THE BUSINESS OF PERSONAL TRAINING

Scott O. Roberts, MS, CSCS
Texas Tech University
Lubbock, Texas

Editor

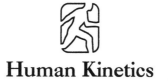

Human Kinetics

Library of Congress Cataloging-in-Publication Data

The business of personal training / Scott O. Roberts, editor.
     p.   cm.
    Includes bibliographical references and index.
    ISBN 0-87322-605-4
    1. Personal trainers. 2. Physical fitness--Vocational guidance.
1. Roberts, Scott.
GV428.7.B87   1996
613.7'11'023--dc20   96-19815
                                           CIP

ISBN-10: 0-87322-605-4
ISBN-13: 978-0-87322-605-9

Acquisitions Editor: Rick Frey, PhD; **Developmental Editor:** Julia Anderson; **Assistant Editors:** Jacqueline Eaton Blakley and Ed Giles; **Copyeditor:** June Waldman; **Proofreader:** Kathy Bennett; **Indexer:** Theresa J. Schaefer; **Typesetting and Layout:** Julie Overholt; **Text Designer:** Robert Reuther; **Photo Editor:** Boyd LaFoon; **Cover Designer:** Keith Blomberg; **Photographer (cover):** Kevin Syms/F-Stock; **Illustrators:** Jennifer Delmotte and Bruce Morton; **Printer:** United Graphics

Printed in the United States of America   10   9   8

Human Kinetics
Web site: www.HumanKinetics.com

United States: Human Kinetics
P.O. Box 5076
Champaign, IL 61825-5076
800-747-4457
e-mail: humank@hkusa.com

Canada: Human Kinetics
475 Devonshire Road Unit 100
Windsor, ON N8Y 2L5
800-465-7301 (in Canada only)
e-mail: orders@hkcanada.com

Europe: Human Kinetics
107 Bradford Road
Stanningley
Leeds LS28 6AT, United Kingdom
+44 (0) 113 255 5665
e-mail: hk@hkeurope.com

Australia: Human Kinetics
57A Price Avenue
Lower Mitcham, South Australia 5062
08 8277 1555
e-mail: liaw@hkaustralia.com

New Zealand: Human Kinetics
Division of Sports Distributors NZ Ltd.
P.O. Box 300 226 Albany
North Shore City
Auckland
0064 9 448 1207
e-mail: info@humankinetics.co.nz

The authors would like to dedicate this book to those individuals who have committed their livelihood to the field of personal training. We can think of no better pursuit in life than to help people improve their health, fitness, and well-being.

Contents

Preface

The purpose of this book is to provide essential information for the professional personal trainer. It focuses on the business aspects of personal training, not on the subject matter of exercise training. Numerous books are available that provide important information and guidelines on how to develop safe and effective exercise programs for clients. A missing resource for personal trainers is a book that tells *how* to become a successful personal trainer.

The Business of Personal Training bridges the gap between the science and theory of personal training and the down-to-earth, practical issues involved in starting and maintaining a successful personal training business. This book contains practical information and advice for personal trainers who want to run a successful business. It includes numerous forms that can be reproduced and strategies from leading personal trainers on how to set up and manage a personal training business.

In Part I of the book, a definition of personal training is followed by a discussion of the origin and evolution of the field. The field of personal training is a new specialty and continues to define itself. Next, the book addresses the qualifications for a personal trainer. Because this is an emerging profession, these qualifications are dynamic and will continue to evolve over the next decade.

In Part II the business side of personal training is covered more completely than in any other publication on personal training. Experienced personal trainers explain the business aspects of personal training, including how to establish a personal training business, how to market and manage a business, and how to meet the legal and professional responsibilities of a personal training business. Part II will help both experienced and new personal trainers understand the business skills necessary to succeed in this dynamic field.

Part III looks at the personal side of personal training. The client–trainer relationship is examined, especially the ethics of this relationship. The psychology of changing the health behaviors of clients is reviewed in depth, and the importance of feedback and motivation are emphasized. Essential and effective communication and teaching techniques for the personal trainer are explained and applied to common situations. Lastly, the chapter on exercise program design summarizes effective ways to help clients achieve their goals.

The Business of Personal Training is a valuable reference for established personal trainers, as well as for those thinking about entering the business. Throughout the book, advice from veteran personal trainers will help the reader appreciate the demands, challenges, and opportunities of this new profession. Ethical and safety considerations in all phases of the client–trainer relationship are addressed throughout the book. Whether you earn $200 per hour or $15 per hour, *The Business of Personal Training* will help you become a more successful personal trainer.

Acknowledgments

I would like to thank the following individuals, who made this book possible:

- The contributors: Mark Reiff, Jack Jones, David Rusk, Amy Huggins, Gregory Florez, David Herbert, Kathy Alexander, Irv Rubenstein, James Gavin, Nettie Gavin, and Douglas Brooks.

- The great people at Human Kinetics, especially Rainer Martens, Rick Frey, and Julia Anderson.
- And especially my family, Andrew, Daniel, Michael, and Julia, for giving me support and encouragement throughout this project.

Credits

Figures 3.1 and 3.2 are from "Survey of Personal Trainers in Houston, Texas" by D.Q. Thomas, K.A. Long, and B. Myers, 1993, *NSCA Journal*, 15(3), p. 43. Copyright 1993 by the National Strength and Conditioning Association. Reprinted by permission.

Figure 3.3 is from *Personal Trainer Certification Brochure* by the National Strength and Conditioning Association, 1993, Lincoln, NE: NSCA. Copyright 1993 by the NSCA. Adapted by permission.

Figure 3.4 is from "Personal Training: State of the Art or State of Neglect" by C. Earnest, 1992, *Conditioning Instructor*, 2(4). Copyright 1992 by the National Strength and Conditioning Association. Adapted by permission.

Figure 3.5 is from *Guidelines for Exercise Testing and Prescription, Fourth Edition* (pp. 240-248) by the American College of Sports Medicine, 1991, Philadelphia: Lea & Febiger. Copyright 1991 by Lea & Febiger. Reprinted by permission.

Figure 7.1 is from *Guidelines for Exercise Testing and Prescription, Fourth Edition* (p. 59) by the American College of Sports Medicine, 1991, Philadelphia: Lea & Febiger. Copyright 1991 by Lea & Febiger. Reprinted by permission.

Figure 7.2 is reprinted in part from the 1994 revised version of the Physical Activity Readiness Questionnaire (PAR-Q and YOU) by special permission from the Canadian Society for Exercise Physiology. Copyright 1994, CSEP.

Figures 7.3 and 7.4 are reprinted with permission from *Legal Aspects of Personal Fitness Training* by B. Koeberle. © Copyright 1990 Professional Reports Corporation, 4418 Belden Village St. N.W., Canton, OH 44718. (800) 336-0083. All Rights Reserved.

Figures 7.5 and 7.6 are from *Essentials of Strength Training and Conditioning* (pp. 498-500 and p. 515) by the National Strength and Conditioning Association, 1994, Champaign, IL: Human Kinetics. Copyright 1994 by the National Strength and Conditioning Association. Reprinted by permission.

Figure 8.1 is from *An Introduction to Borg's RPE-Scale* by G. Borg, 1985, Ithaca, NY: Mouvement Publications. Copyright 1985 by Gunnar Borg. Reprinted by permission.

Figures 9.2 and 9.3 are from *Psychology for Health Fitness Professionals* (p. 43 and p. 76) by J. Gavin and N. Gavin, 1995, Champaign, IL: Human Kinetics. Copyright 1995 by James Gavin and Nettie Gavin. Reprinted by permission.

Figure 10.1 is from *The Interpersonal Communication Book* (6th ed., p. 55) by Joseph A. DeVito, 1992, New York: HarperCollins. Copyright © 1992 by Joseph A. DeVito. Reprinted by permission of HarperCollins Publishers, Inc.

Table 10.1 is from *The Art of Communication* by B. Decker, 1988, Los Altos, CA: Crisp. Copyright 1988 by Crisp Publications, Inc., 1200 Hamilton Court, Menlo Park, CA 94025; 800-442-7477. Adapted by permission.

Table 10.2 is from *Listening Made Easy* by R.L. Montgomery, 1981, New York: AMACOM. Copyright 1981 by Robert L. Montgomery. Adapted by permission.

Figure 11.1 is from *Going Solo: The Art of Personal Training* (p. 120) by D.S. Brooks, 1990, Mammoth Lakes, CA: Moves International. Reprinted by permission.

Table 11.1 is from *Weight Training: Steps to Success* (p.146) by T. Baechle and B. Groves, 1992, Champaign, IL: Human Kinetics. Copyright 1992 by Leisure Press. Adapted by permission.

Information in the Appendix is from *Fitness Management*, 1995, **11**(3). Copyright 1995 by Leisure Publications, Inc. Reprinted by permission.

Photos

Part II and chapters 3 and 5 opening photos © Mary Langenfeld.

Part III and chapters 1 and 9 opening photos © CLEO Photography.

Chapter 2 opening photo © Bettmann/Marci Brennan.

Chapters 4 and 10 opening photos © Terry Wild Studio.

Chapters 6 and 11 opening photos courtesy of the Shiley Sports and Health Center of Scripps Clinic and Research Foundation.

Chapter 7 opening photo © Cheyenne Rouse.

Part I
Personal Training as a Profession

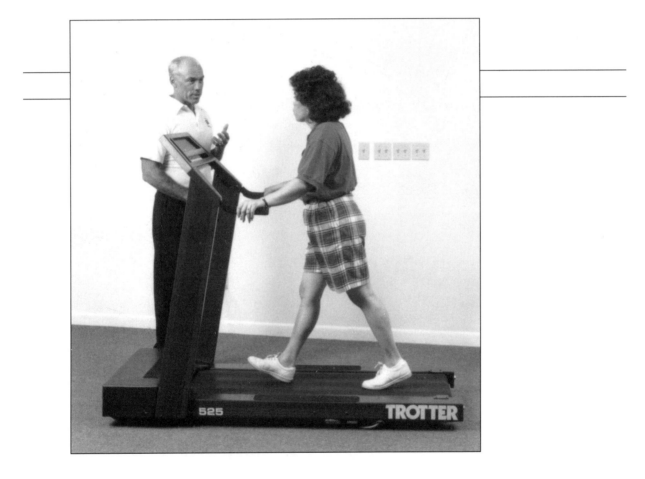

As stated in the preface, the purpose of this book is to provide essential information about the profession of personal training. Before discussing how to become a successful personal trainer, it is important to define personal training. If you don't already know what a personal trainer does, the title alone will give you a clue about the work of a personal trainer. The word *training* implies some kind of teacher or educator role. A personal trainer must be involved in teaching, or training, people how to do something. What about the word *personal*? A personal trainer must be involved in working with people on an individual or very personal level. Thus, a *personal trainer* is someone who teaches individuals how to do something, usually on an individual level. Well then, a music teacher, a golf pro, or a football coach could all be considered personal trainers. Why the field of fitness was given the privilege of using the term *personal trainer* to describe someone who works with individuals one-on-one to help them get in shape, no one will ever know for sure. Nevertheless, the term *personal training* is now firmly embedded in the health and fitness industry.

So then, how do fitness professionals define personal training? Although there really is no official or legal definition of personal training, Mark Reiff provides a reasonable explanation and definition in chapter 1. After you read chapter 1, you will realize that the current definition of personal training is quite broad. A personal trainer is an educator, motivator, business person, nutritionist, psychologist, coach, exercise physiologist, and more! With time, or with state or federal licensure, personal training may take on a more formal definition.

Of even more interest than the definition of personal training is the development of the personal training field. In chapter 2, Jack Jones presents an excellent historical overview of the emergence of the personal training field. As the author states, "Surely personal training has been with us, in some form or other, since humans started competing in sports." Although we will probably never know the exact origin of personal fitness training, it has evolved into a respectable and growing field. In fact, there are even some health clubs that exclusively offer one-on-one training.

So you want to become a personal trainer—where do you go to learn the trade? As you will see by reading the biographies of the authors of this book and by talking with other personal trainers, personal trainers have diverse backgrounds. Chapter 3 presents a recent survey of personal trainers that sheds some light on their qualifications and training. In reality, the more training and education personal trainers have, the more likely it is that they will be successful.

Chapter 1

Defining Personal Training

Mark A. Reiff

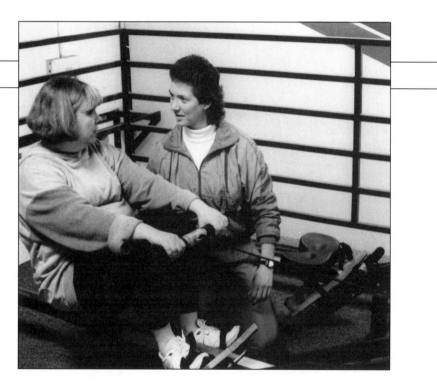

The objectives of this chapter are to

- define personal training and
- describe the characteristics of a good personal trainer.

Overview

This chapter attempts to define personal training. The definition of a field or profession is usually based on a formal job description. Because the field of personal training is so new, job descriptions vary greatly from one facility or business to the next. Without a standardized job description, defining personal training is rather difficult. Personal trainers who work for a health club may only be required to train clients; those who own and operate their own business must perform a variety of additional functions, including marketing and bookkeeping. Personal fitness training can be broadly defined as a profession that employs qualified individuals to instruct and train clients, usually in a one-on-one situation, in the performance of safe and appropriate exercise, in an effort to achieve the clients' personal fitness and health goals.

The age-old adage about a profession being half art and half science is nowhere truer than in personal training. Although there is still a lot of art involved in personal training, a recent explosion of scientific knowledge about the body and how it responds and adapts to exercise has taken place in recent years and shifted the balance toward the science side of the scale. The body of knowledge that has accumulated over the last two decades about physical and mental conditioning is truly astounding. As recently as the mid-1950s, the only people who indulged in strength training using weights were body builders and power lifters; coaches and trainers actually forbade football, basketball, and baseball players to lift weights on the grounds that they would become "muscle-bound." In those days, the theory was that muscle development would slow the athlete's reaction time, reduce flexibility, and impair coordination.

Of course, those were also the days when enduring a 2-hour conditioning workout without water was supposed to develop a mentally tough, determined athlete—and when the duck waddle that probably ruined a couple of generations of knees was a common exercise for football conditioning. As recently as the mid-1960s, cross-country runners who attached water bottles to their belts would have been laughed off the road. The reason for all the misinformation coaches purveyed in those unenlightened days was simply lack of information. Early coaches formulated their methods and philosophies from various combinations of their own participation and training in a sport, informal observations, whatever reading they might do on the subject (and there wasn't much), and trial and error. Some coaches, though by no means all, fine-tuned their knowledge and passed on to younger athletes better information than they themselves initially received. Through this evolution of knowledge, the field of personal training was born.

What Is Personal Training?

The field of personal training is relatively new. Today's personal trainers, whether they are in business for themselves or employed by clubs or corporations, must be jacks-of-all-trades in order to do well. Successful personal trainers learned early on that the field was not based simply on physical conditioning. Besides the obvious preparation needed to become a competent personal trainer, individuals who want to succeed in personal training as a career or business will need to prepare themselves to be competent businesspeople, motivators, and teachers. Besides

knowing how to train a client, personal trainers need to know how to create, market, and manage a business. The definition of personal training is broad and multifaceted. Personal trainers can expect to perform a variety of functions during the course of their career. Individuals entering the field of personal training will need to prepare themselves in a variety of areas (see Table 1.1).

For the most part, personal training today means a client working with a personal trainer in a one-on-one situation. People hire personal trainers for many reasons, including the need for specialized care when recovering from an illness or accident, the commitment to improve their fitness level, and probably the most common reason is the desire to have someone to motivate and educate them. Personal training clients come from all walks of life. Some are models or movie stars, some are professional athletes whose careers depend on how well they perform, and a large percentage are average people. Whatever their reasons for wanting a personal trainer, however, almost everyone wants a personal trainer who is highly qualified.

Personal trainers might have a degree from a 2- or 4-year college, or not. They may be certified by one of several fitness organizations, or not. Some trainers have simply learned a lot about personal training and exercise on their own. Whatever the formal training, the first requirement for a personal trainer is understanding the field. This means developing a detailed knowledge of anatomy, physiology, and kinesiology (the study of movement); a thorough understanding of the prevention and treatment of exercise-related injury; an understanding of the psychological aspects of training; and knowledge of how to start and manage a business. In addition to these basic skills, good trainers must understand how to motivate people if they want to keep their clients interested and progressing toward their goals. Personal trainers also need to know about nutrition and proper eating habits, weight loss and gain, and dietary fads. In essence,

Table 1.1 Components of Personal Training

Marketing	Legal responsibilities
Business structures	Management
Psychology	Education
Communicating	Ethics and professional
Teaching	responsibilities
Professional preparation	Certification
Understanding of the field	Program design
of personal training	Safety

personal trainers need to be prepared to perform many job functions.

An important measure of a personal trainer's qualifications is certification. Personal training clients are knowledgeable consumers and frequently ask personal trainers what kind of certification they have. When personal trainers have a certification from a nonaccredited or fly-by-night organization, today's fitness consumer may not be satisfied. Fitness professionals can select from a variety of professional certifications. The following organizations offer certification in personal training: National Strength and Conditioning Association (NSCA), American College of Sports Medicine (ACSM), American Council on Exercise (ACE), Aerobics and Fitness Association of America (AFAA), International Association for Fitness Professionals (IDEA), Canadian Society of Exercise Physiology (CSEP). Today's personal trainer should obtain professional certification from at least one respected certifying agency.

The purpose of this book is to help personal trainers become better personal trainers and to learn new skills necessary for success in the field. However, this is not the only book personal trainers need to read in order to be successful. All personal trainers should be well versed in a variety of subjects. It is important to remember that individuals who succeed at personal training have to prepare themselves to perform a variety of functions.

The Personal Side of Personal Training

Because personal trainers must deal with everyone— from the self-conscious client who knows little and is almost embarrassed to be working out to the expert fitness buff—they must excel in what have become known as *people skills*. Good people skills cannot be learned simply by reading a book. Communication and teaching skills need to be practiced with a diverse group of people and in a variety of situations. How you communicate with one person may be completely different from how you communicate with another person. Developing good people skills is an essential skill personal trainers must learn, apply, and practice daily.

Most trainers find that the most difficult clients are the ones who actually understand very little about how the body works, but who have picked up just enough jargon to be dangerous. Much folklore has crept into physical conditioning over the years, and many myths are accepted as fact. The personal trainer must at least try to reeducate clients who believe those myths.

Trainers must also know how to talk with clients because trainers need to analyze, or at least relate to, their clients' personalities. Often clients are as interested in talking as they are in working out; the trainer's skill in this area goes a long way in determining the best way to train each client. Personal trainers need to know when to make a client really work up a sweat and when to slow down. Trainers must learn how to talk; how to listen; how to keep themselves from playing psychiatrist when the impulse to do so is overwhelming; and how to encourage, encourage, and encourage some more.

Part III of this book shows you how to become better at communicating with your client, by focusing on the client–trainer relationship, the psychology of personal training, communication and training techniques, and designing individual exercise programs. Your relationship with a client is special and unique. Relationships take time to develop, and the personal trainer–client relationship is no different. Individuals who succeed at personal training are generally good at communicating with other individuals.

The Business Side of Personal Training

Whether in a club or in their own gym, trainers must also understand business. That means marketing and sales; it means knowing how to set prices and collect fees; it means staying abreast of rules, regulations, and the tax laws; it means understanding Social Security and unemployment taxes; and it means basic bookkeeping.

Some trainers feel that the most important aspect of personal training is how knowledgeable they are about the body and how well they show their concern for clients. Over time, successful personal trainers come to understand that unless they know how to sell their services and how to run a business, the rest of their knowledge is not worth much.

Frequently, clubs display pictures of the "Trainer of the Month." Members may think the selection is based on knowledge, training techniques, a winning personality, or sincerity, but trainers know better: The award is often based on the month's sales figures. The interesting thing is that when trainers excel at what they do and genuinely love it, they often turn out to be good salespeople for fitness too.

Learning essential business skills is important to the success of any business, whether large or small. Selected chapters in this book discuss how to create, manage, and market your personal training business, as well as the legal and professional responsibilities of personal trainers. There are lots of personal trainers who have never considered that they are in a business. Perhaps they never thought about going out on their own or about choosing personal training as their career. Individuals who succeed at personal training are generally good businesspeople.

Summary

The field of personal training is a relatively new field that is rapidly growing in popularity. In the past, few personal trainers ever expected to make a living at personal training. Perhaps it was a way to get through college or a way to earn some extra income. Today it is possible to earn a good, even great, living as a personal trainer. To be a successful personal trainer, you must be prepared to perform a variety of roles. In addition to being a good one-on-one communicator, you must develop good business skills.

Chapter 2

The Origin of Personal Training

Jack Jones

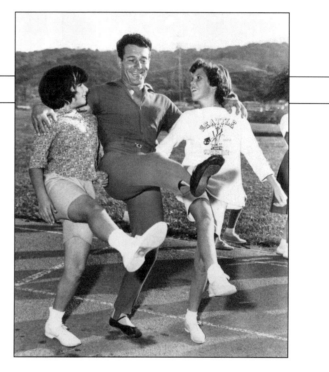

The objectives of this chapter are to

- review the brief history of personal training,
- review the role of the club-based personal trainer, and
- discuss the backgrounds of personal trainers.

Overview

It is difficult to determine exactly where and when the field of personal training actually started. One could argue that personal training began on Venice Beach or in a fancy health club or maybe in a movie star's home in Beverly Hills. Regardless of its exact origin, personal training has emerged as a prominent profession, affecting millions of fitness and health consumers. More than likely, the profession arose from a luxury once only affluent consumers could afford. Today most fitness consumers can find personal trainers within their budget. Walk into any health club today, and you will probably find personal training services available. The field of personal training has dramatically changed the way people exercise and has probably increased the percentage of Americans who start and stay with an exercise program.

In 1993 a Greek vase was discovered depicting athletes about to begin a foot race. There was nothing particularly unusual about the discovery except that on this vase, standing behind the runners, is someone who appears to be a race official holding the end of a rope against which the runners are leaning. The rope is apparently the ancient Greek version of the starting pistol. What doesn't show, on that vase or in the pages of history books, are the runners' trainers.

Yet surely personal training has been with us, in some form or other, since human beings started competing in sports. I can't believe there wasn't an archer somewhere in Switzerland who didn't seek out William Tell for advice on arrows or someone in Merrie Olde England who didn't plead with Robin Hood for tips on shooting. Back in the American Wild West, wouldn't some up-and-coming young gunslinger have sought out Wyatt Earp or Doc Holiday for a few pointers? Could anyone imagine Japan's samurai not having personal trainers? We'll probably never know who the earliest personal trainers were, or how they operated, although we do see an athlete hire a personal trainer in the movie *Chariots of Fire*, which was supposed to have taken place in 1920s England.

The History of Personal Training

Until well into this century, the great majority of ordinary people did such hard physical labor—farming, factory jobs, mining, construction, and road work, for instance—that few people needed extra exercise to stay fit. My guess is that personal training began among the affluent, as soon as people with a little leisure time decided they wanted to excel in individual athletic endeavors—whether that sport was archery, tennis, or golf. At the same time, personal trainers probably began teaching specific team-sports skills, such as shooting a basketball, passing a football, and pitching and hitting a baseball.

During the 1930s, there was some interest in resistance exercises and weightlifting (or body building as it was then called), with brothers Ben and Joe Weider laying the foundation for body building as a competitive sport. The Weider brothers were among the first to promote building muscle for its own sake, rather than as a means to excel in a particular sport. The organizations and contests they created to publicize body building indirectly created another avenue for personal trainers. The Weiders are considered pioneers in body building (see Figure 2.1).

It was only after the country began its economic recovery from World War II that the general public slowly began to be interested in nutrition and health and to look for ways to find out more about these areas. The body of knowledge about how physical fitness could be achieved was still very limited and remained so until well into the 1970s. Those were the days when coaches fed athletes salt tablets, withheld water during practice sessions, and were opposed to resistance exercises on the ground that it made athletes muscle-bound.

Pioneers in Personal Training

The earliest health clubs designed for the general public were probably the ones started back in 1947 when Vic Tanny opened an exercise facility in a Second Street loft in Santa Monica, California. By 1961, Tanny owned more than 100 such clubs, from Los Angeles to Chicago to New York City and was reportedly earning several million dollars a year. Because success breeds competition, Tanny was not alone in the health club business for very long. From 1947 to the present, the number of clubs and the number of personal trainers has grown exponentially.

So, fortunately, has the state of knowledge about fitness and how to achieve and maintain it. Over the past few years, the body of information about what it takes to keep the human body in top form has grown so quickly that it is difficult for professionals to keep abreast of new developments. The demand for personal trainers began during the early 1950s and grew very slowly over the next 20 years. At about the time Vic Tanny was beginning his business in Santa Monica, a few other pioneers were also entering the field in a variety of ways. The effect these people had in exposing the public to the idea of exercise and fitness raised general awareness of the benefits of health clubs—and eventually, convinced many people to hire personal trainers to help them meet their fitness goals.

Some of these early pioneers were personal trainers and club owners. Others, not all of them trainers themselves, were advocates of group exercise who developed television exercise shows, and later, fitness videos. Jack LaLanne, for example, began his fitness career in the 1950s and for many years starred in a television exercise show originating in San Francisco. (Bette Davis once commented that she frequently exercised to Jack LaLanne's program.)

Another pioneer of the 1950s, Ray Wilson, bought existing health clubs and built new ones to establish

1930s	Interest in resistance exercises and weightlifting began. Brothers Ben and Joe Weider established body building as a competitive sport.
1940s	After the end of World War II, the general public slowly began to be interested in nutrition and health.
1947	Vic Tanny opened an exercise facility in a Second Street loft in Santa Monica, California.
1950s	The demand for personal trainers began. At about the time Vic Tanny was beginning his business in Santa Monica, a few other pioneers were also entering the field. Jack LaLanne's fitness television show began in San Francisco. Ray Wilson bought established health clubs and built new ones to establish his American Health Club.
1960s	Dr. Kenneth Cooper's books popularized the term *aerobic exercise*.
1970s	Jackie Sorensen turned aerobic dance into a business. Ten years later, after conducting workshops and demonstrations nationwide, her business had grown to some 180,000 students and 4,000 instructors. Many celebrities became fitness advocates. Jake Steinfeld introduced his rough, tough "Body by Jake" fitness routine.
1980s	By the 1980s, many people were ready to get serious about regular exercise and began to join health clubs and hire personal trainers.
1990s	Several organizations offer certification programs for personal trainers. Major conferences focus on the business of personal trainers. Most health clubs offer some type of personal training service.

Figure 2.1 Evolution of personal training.

his American Health Club and Family Fitness chain. In the late 1950s, Dr. Kenneth Cooper came on the scene. Dr. Cooper, one of the giants of the health and fitness field, has written many fitness books and brought the term *aerobic exercise* into common use; he still maintains a well-respected health and exercise research center in Dallas, Texas. In the early 1970s, Jackie Sorensen was one of the first to enter the aerobic dance business. Ten years later, after conducting workshops and demonstrations nationwide, her business had grown to some 180,000 students and 4,000 instructors. The "Joy of Movement" club in the Boston area, originally started as a dance studio, was another early entrant in the aerobic dance and fitness field.

The 1970s also saw the beginning of the trend for movie stars to become advocates of fitness, among them Christopher Reeve, who played Superman, and Arnold Schwarzenegger; they were followed in the 1980s by Cher, Madonna, and other celebrities. Jane Fonda was the first movie star to produce exercise videos specifically designed for people who wanted to work out privately at home. Fonda even targeted specific exercise videos to specific kinds of clients, such as pregnant women. Jake Steinfeld, with his rough, tough "Body by Jake" presentation also became prominent in the 1970s as a trainer of movie

stars. With his television program and books on fitness, Steinfeld is still a prominent figure in the field.

By the 1980s, thanks to all these factors and others (including a burgeoning interest in proper nutrition and lowering the amount of dietary fat), many people were ready to get serious about regular exercise. Many fledgling exercisers began to join health clubs and hire personal trainers.

Personal Trainers Emerging in Health Clubs

Initially, the primary job of health-club–based personal trainers was to sell club memberships and to teach new members how to use the equipment. After those functions had been fulfilled, they were free to recruit personal clients from among the ranks of the club's membership, through other contacts, or both. Most of these trainers were paid solely on a commission basis for the memberships they sold and either by commission or fees from their personal training clients. This arrangement led to most clubs having three groups of trainers. The first group, naturally most valued by club owners, were those who were good at both training and selling. The second group included those who were good sellers but not-so-good trainers, and the third group included those who were good trainers but not good salespeople. Those in group three were usually fired, leaving clubs with a large group of people who were good sellers but not-so-good trainers. This worked out fine for club owners, but not so well for clients, and tarnished reputations of the better trainers and the entire personal training field.

Today, most personal trainers who work in better health clubs are not expected to double as salespeople. Their functions, status, and remuneration are so varied and complex, even within the same group of franchises, that it is hard to describe them simply. For instance, some clubs hire personal trainers as staff members and pay them a small wage; their primary functions are to help new members develop workout programs and to answer questions from people working out on the floor. These trainers may also recruit personal clients, but the club typically determines and collects the fees the trainers receive from their personal clients, paying the trainer an hourly rate for training sessions that is somewhat higher than the rate they are paid for "working the floor."

Other clubs use personal trainers who are independent contractors. Some of these contractors pay the club a fixed fee for the use of their facilities. In other cases, each trainer determines how much his or her personal clients will pay and may then pay a percentage of the fee to the club. Under the latter arrangement, the club usually expects the independent contractor–trainers to help on the floor as well, in exchange for the privilege of "farming" the membership for new personal clients.

From the 1940s until well into the 1980s, most personal trainers had little or no formal education in teaching or exercise physiology. Since most of them learned what they knew from other trainers, misinformation and ineffective methods were perpetuated, and very little was written about physical conditioning. In spite of all these problems, the public's willingness to pay for personal training has grown, and the competence level of personal trainers has increased. Today, the quality and status of personal trainers vary with geographical location, the type of club (public or private), and employment arrangements. Geographically, personal trainers are more in demand in southern California than in most other regions of the country; there are also more personal trainers in large urban areas than elsewhere; and private clubs usually offer better trainers because they pay them more.

However, it is nearly impossible for trainers to earn enough money to survive solely on what they earn

in most public health clubs, and most of them work in clubs only part-time. This creates high staff turnover. I worked for a large public chain in Los Angeles for a year, and at any one time, there were between 10 and 15 trainers on staff. Over the course of that year, more than 100 different trainers passed through the club.

A few trainers manage to become financially independent through running private consulting businesses, although this is the most difficult road to travel because it requires the time and knowledge to handle advertising and promotion, networking, bookkeeping, and all the other aspects of running a successful small business. As the proliferation of health and fitness clubs has continued, the demand for qualified personal trainers has grown, at first slowly and then quickly. Currently, there is very strong demand.

The Need to Certify Trainer Competence

In the early days, physical education teachers, coaches, and former athletes were the only pool from which clubs could hire qualified trainers. When the demand exceeded the number of truly qualified trainers, clubs responded by downgrading their requirements. That imbalance has constantly become more pronounced, opening the floodgates of the unqualified. The result has been a large number of less qualified, lower paid, and less professional trainers.

Competence is as necessary for personal trainers as it is for doctors, nurses, and therapists, because trainers are responsible for providing correct information to people who are trying to develop and maintain health and fitness. Personal trainers, like other professionals, are specialists. As the body of knowledge about fitness continues to grow, it will be even more important that the people conveying that information are qualified to do so.

The skill level of the personal trainers working in health clubs today ranges from excellent to incompetent, with the majority, unfortunately, at the lower end of the scale. (The best trainers often try a few clubs and then move out to start their own business.) Fortunately, however, as the public has become better informed about fitness, diet, and exercise, its ability to spot incompetent trainers has increased. As more people have become more discerning, more members are complaining to club managers about incompetent trainers and demanding better ones—or leaving to join other clubs. This, of course, benefits both the public and the personal training profession.

The need to attain and maintain some level of credibility for trainers has resulted in some colleges and universities instituting certification programs. Certification examinations for a variety of positions related to health and fitness have also been devised. In 1982 the American College of Sports Medicine (ACSM) was among the first organizations to respond to the need to upgrade the quality of personal trainers. The ACSM developed and published guidelines and written examinations for personal trainers and five other areas of health, fitness, and aerobic instruction. As of September 1993, ACSM had certified 6,000 people in these six areas.

In 1986 the American Council on Exercise (ACE) began certification programs and examinations for aerobics instructors and personal trainers. As of September 1993, ACE had certified 19,000 aerobics instructors and 6,000 personal trainers. The National Strength and Conditioning Association (NSCA) has developed a certification program for Certified Strength and Conditioning Specialists (CSCS) and plans to offer personal training certification as well. Other organizations, such as the Aerobics and Fitness Association of America (AFAA), offer certifications also. In Canada, the Canadian Society for Exercise Physiology (CSEP) offers a program for Certified Fitness Appraisers (CFA).

At present, ACSM and ACE seem to be the most respected certification organizations. In spite of all this activity, however, there is no single agency that examines and approves or ranks certification examinations. The National Organization of Competency Assurance (1101 Connecticut Avenue NW, Suite 700, Washington, DC 20036), will examine documents from an organization and make a judgment about quality, but the association has no ranking system. Like professionals in any field, good personal trainers welcome efforts to improve both the competence and the degree of respect accorded to their ranks. It is a hopeful sign that so much is happening to bring this about.

Summary

The field of personal training has emerged as a respected profession. With its roots embedded in the early foundations of physical fitness and weight training, personal trainers today are required to possess a wide range of skills and talents. Today most health clubs in American hire personal trainers. Fitness consumers also hire personal trainers to come to their homes and offices. This is an exciting period in the evolution of the personal training field. Personal training has created thousands of job opportunities for health, physical education, and exercise science graduates. Personal training may very well be the way of the future when it comes to exercise. No longer are movie stars the only employers of personal trainers. Personal trainers are now integrated into all aspects of the fitness industry.

Note: I am indebted to Sam Calhoun, one of the "Muscle Beach Originals," for much of the early California history related in this chapter. Sam has made fitness training his career for more than 30 years and is certified by the American College of Sports Medicine as Fitness Instructor, Graded Exercise Test Technologist, and Exercise Specialist.

Chapter 3

Qualifications for Personal Training

Scott O. Roberts

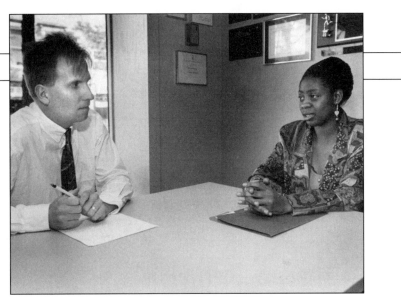

The objectives of this chapter are to

- review different opinions regarding the qualifications needed to be a personal trainer,
- review a survey of personal trainer qualifications, and
- review the certification standards of several different professional associations.

Overview

There are no universal or minimum qualifications needed to call yourself a personal trainer. Until such time personal trainers are required to become licensed, qualifications will continue to vary greatly. Different professional certifications require minimum qualifications, for example, a college degree, CPR certification, or a certain number of practicum hours. If your goal is to work for a health club or company that requires a specific certification, then the minimum qualifications you need to be a personal trainer are the qualifications required to take that particular certification. Personal trainers come from many backgrounds, with diverse education and training preparation. Personal trainers are lawyers, accountants, coaches, and exercise enthusiasts, as well as exercise physiologists and physical education teachers. In the coming years colleges may start offering degrees in personal training. Until such time, most personal trainers will obtain their education and training from a variety of sources. Licensure of personal trainers, similar to licensure of physical therapists or athletic trainers, may still be years away. A good motto for personal trainers to follow regarding training and education is "the more the better." Remember, most personal trainers perform a variety of functions, including psychologist, medical expert, coach, exercise physiologist, weight loss expert, and accountant, and need to be informed in all these areas.

Personal trainers offer instruction and advice to clients on exercise, as well as other areas of personal health, such as nutrition and wellness. The personal training business has evolved from a luxury that only those with significant economic resources could afford to a privilege now available to a much broader segment of the population (Brooks, 1990). The evolution of the personal training field has resulted in personal trainers with highly variable, nonstandardized qualifications. Because the fitness industry is relatively unregulated, personal trainers are generally held to standards developed by professional associations. Certification from a nationally recognized professional organization, as well as good documentation of training, education and experience, will enhance the marketability and respect of personal trainers and help protect them in legal matters. This chapter will explore some of the essential qualifications required to be a personal trainer.

Survey of Personal Trainer Qualifications

Personal trainers come from all walks of life. For example, David Rusk, one of the authors of this book, was a successful certified public accountant before he decided to become a personal trainer. There really are no absolute qualifications needed to become a personal trainer. Some states are investigating whether or not personal trainers and aerobic instructors should be licensed, but until a state or national license is required, minimum qualifications or standards required to call oneself a personal trainer are not well defined. At this point, national fitness organizations are primarily responsible for mandating basic competencies and qualifications for personal trainers.

To get some idea of the qualifications of personal trainers, Thomas, Long, and Meyers (1993) recently published a survey of 58 personal trainers in Houston, Texas (see Figure 3.1). Of the 58 respondents, 62% were male and 38% were female. Forty-two percent of the respondents had over 6 years experience; only 1 participant had less than 1 year of experience. Eight-four percent reported attending an institute of higher education, with 62% earning a bachelor's degree or above. Ten percent reported earning a master's degree, and 41% earned degrees in exercise science or a related field. Seventy-one percent of the respondents were certified as a fitness leader, aerobics instructor, or personal trainer.

The results of this survey demonstrate the high degree of variance in training, education, and experience among personal trainers (see Figure 3.2). In the absence of any state or federal regulation of personal trainers, if a personal trainer's actions are challenged in a court of law, expert testimony will be used to determine whether the standard of care was met, and whether the trainer's actions were reasonable, prudent, and consistent with policies and procedures in similar facilities. Ultimately, it is the responsibility of the client to seek out a qualified personal trainer. Personal trainers should expect today's consumer to be knowledgeable when choosing a personal trainer. Consumers need to ask prospective trainers questions such as, what is your education level, what kind of training and preparation do you have, and what certification do you hold?

The Call for Certification

According to the *Random House Dictionary, certified* means "having or proved by a certificate." *Certificate* is defined as "a document attesting to the fact that a person has completed an educational course or test of knowledge." Each organization that offers certification will define the parameters of that certification. Basically certification as a personal trainer is a standard by which certain skills and knowledge are viewed and measured. Certification does not imply competency in any areas not specifically and clearly outlined in the behavioral objectives of the required examination(s).

Several fitness associations have developed personal trainer examinations, including the National Strength and Conditioning Association, the Cooper Institute for Aerobics Research, the American College of Sports Medicine, the American Council on Exercise, the Aerobics and Fitness Association of America, and the Canadian Society of Exercise Physiology.

1. How many years have you been a personal trainer?
   A. Less than 1
   B. 1-3
   C. 4-5
   D. 6-7
   E. 8-10
   F. More than 10

2. Were you a varsity athlete?   Yes   No
   A. If yes, at what level?
      1. Professional
      2. College
      3. High school
      4. Other
   B. In what sport?
      1. Football
      2. Track and field
      3. Basketball
      4. Baseball
      5. Volleyball
      6. Hockey
      7. Other

3. Do you have a college degree?   Yes   No
   A. If yes, what degree?
      1. Associate
      2. Bachelor's
      3. Master's
      4. Doctoral
   B. In what area?
      1. Exercise science
      2. Business
      3. Other

4. What type of institution did you attend?
   A. Junior/community college
   B. College
   C. University
   D. Did not attend higher education

5. Do you hold any certifications   Yes   No
   A. If yes, what certifications?
      1. First aid
      2. CPR
      3. Fitness instructor
      4. Other

6. Have you successfully completed a college course in:
   A. Nutrition
   B. Anatomy
   C. Physiology
   D. Exercise physiology
   E. Biochemistry
   F. Biomechanics/kinesiology
   G. Exercise prescription
   H. Fitness programming
   I. Weight training and conditioning
   J. Sports medicine

7. What percentage of the diet should be comprised of protein?
   A. 0-7
   B. 8-15
   C. 16-25
   D. 26-35
   E. More than 35
   F. Don't know

8. What do you recommend as the best way to lose body fat?

9. Do you work out?   Yes   No
   A. If yes, how many times per week
      1. 1
      2. 2
      3. 3
      4. 4
      5. 5
      6. More than 5 days per week
   B. What type of exercise do you perform?
      1. Weight training
      2. Aerobics
      3. Walking
      4. Jogging
      5. Cycling
      6. Swimming
      7. Other
   C. How long does your typical workout last?
      1. 0-10 minutes
      2. 11-20 minutes
      3. 21-30 minutes
      4. 31-40 minutes
      5. 41-50 minutes
      6. 51-60 minutes
      7. Other

10. What is the recommended target zone for someone to work out at to maintain or improve cardiovascular fitness?

Figure 3.1   Personal trainer survey.
Reprinted from Thomas, Long, and Myers (1993).

Years as a personal trainer			Highest level of athletic achievement			Sports participated in by personal trainers*		
>10	9	(16)	Olympic	2	(3)	Track	21	(36)
8-10	3	(5)	Professional	4	(7)	Football	18	(31)
6-7	12	(21)	Semi-pro	1	(2)	Baseball	11	(19)
4-5	9	(16)	College	13	(22)	Basketball	7	(12)
1-3	24	(41)	High school	26	(45)	Volleyball	6	(10)
<1	1	(2)	Nonathlete	12	(21)	Soccer	4	(7)
						Swimming	4	(7)
						Cheerleading	3	(5)
						Other	12	(21)

Data presented as total number of respondents (percentage of total group).
*In some cases, respondents were active in more than one sport.

Type of institution attended			Highest advanced degree earned			Major	
University	35	(60)	Master's	6	(10)	Exercise science	23
College	6	(10)	Bachelor's	30	(52)	Business	5
Junior college	5	(9)	Associate	1	(2)	Communication	3
Other	3	(5)	None	21	(36)	Health	1
						Medical technology	1
						Spanish	1
						English	1
						Hotel management	1
						Dance	1
						Marketing	1
						World literature	1
						Psychology	1

Data presented as total number of respondents (percentage of total group).

Figure 3.2 Experience and educational background of personal trainers.
Reprinted from Thomas, Long, and Myers (1993).

Generally, certifications are developed after extensive analysis and research into the specific responsibilities of personal trainers. An organization begins by assembling a panel of experts that outlines the key areas of a personal trainer's responsibilities, sometimes referred to as *core tasks*. Next, a survey is sent out to hundreds of fitness professionals who comment on the various items included in the inventory of core tasks. After the responses are collected and analyzed, the organization asks another group of professionals to write test questions. This process is sometimes referred to as *item writing*. Then, the sample questions are verified for accuracy and rated on how well they reflect the core tasks previously identified. Finally, the examination is printed. Figure 3.3 lists NSCA's Certified Personal Trainer Job Analysis Task List (NSCA, 1993). This list was compiled by a group of experts in an effort to design a certification that would accurately test all the skills required for personal trainers. Think of the job analysis task list

as a sample job description for a personal trainer. It can help you determine your strengths and weaknesses as a personal trainer, as well as help you prepare for the NSCA's personal trainer exam.

As you can see, developing a certification is not an easy task. Figure 3.4 (p. 19) lists the nationally recognized personal trainer certifications. Take a look at each one and decide which certification you may want to hold. (It certainly doesn't hurt to have more than one certification.) You might want to send for information on all of them before deciding which is best for you. Another good way to decide on the best certification for you is to talk with other personal trainers and health club managers and owners.

What qualifications are important in becoming a personal trainer? Based on the responses of some of the top fitness experts in the country, several general areas stand out regarding professional preparation, experience, and certification for personal trainers. First, some minimal level of education is desired.

I. Client Consultation/Assessment

    A.   Initial Interview
        1. Determine client–trainer compatibility
        2. Determine client goals
        3. Complete client–trainer agreement
        4. Complete informed consent and waiver form

    B.   Health Appraisal/Medical History Review
        1. Administer medical history form
        2. Evaluate exercise history (past/present)
        3. Evaluate and interpret results
        4. Recognize those needing referral to appropriate health care professional

    C.   Fitness Evaluation
        1. Conduct fitness profile, i.e., vital signs (heart rate, blood pressure), body composition, etc.
        2. Evaluate and interpret results
        3. Recognize clients needing referral to appropriate health care professional

    D.   Basic Nutrition and Weight Management
        1. Evaluate current nutritional status
        2. Evaluate current dietary habits
        3. Recognize eating disorders and make referral to appropriate health care professional

II. Program Planning

    A.   Goal Setting
        1. Discuss assessment results with client and establish health/fitness program
        2. Prepare schedule for exercise program
        3. Discuss nutritional habits
        4. Motivational techniques (reinforcement strategies)

    B.   Program Design
        1. Select modality (exercise type)
        2. Establish order of exercise components
        3. Establish intensity
        4. Establish duration
        5. Establish frequency
        6. Determine rate of progression

    C.   Recognize Training Outcomes
        1. Neurological
        2. Connective tissue (muscle, tendon, ligament)
        3. Skeletal (bone and cartilage)
        4. Cardiovascular
        5. Metabolic
        6. Psychological changes

    D.   Special Populations
        1. Determine capacities and limitations of special populations, i.e., obese individuals, the elderly, etc.
        2. Modify program to coincide with limitation and capacities of special populations

III. Techniques of Exercise

    A.   Instruct clients on proper use of the following equipment
        1. Resistance machines (weight, hydraulic, air, friction, tubing, etc.)

(continued)

Figure 3.3 NSCA-certified personal trainer job analysis task list.
Adapted from National Strength and Conditioning Association (1993).

---

        a. preparatory body position (grip, stance, etc.)
        b. execution techniques
        c. practice proper spotting techniques
    2. Free weights
        a. preparatory body position (grip, stance, etc.)
        b. execution techniques
        c. practice proper spotting techniques
    3. Cardiovascular machines (treadmills, stair climbers, stationary bikes, rowing, etc.)

  B. Instruct clients on other nonmachine exercise techniques
    1. Cardiovascular (running, walking, etc.)
    2. Flexibility
    3. Calisthenics
    4. Plyometrics (speed, strength, etc.)

IV. Safety, Emergency Procedures, and Legal Issues

  A. Practice Safety Procedures
    1. Recognize properly maintained equipment
    2. Provide a safe exercise environment
    3. Recognize overuse symptoms

  B. Administer Emergency Procedures
    1. First aid
    2. CPR

  C. Recognize Professional, Legal and Ethical Issues
    1. Recognize litigation issues
    2. Maintain client confidentiality
    3. Maintain professional client–trainer relationship
    4. Maintain liability insurance
    5. Practice business and management techniques

Figure 3.3   *(continued)*

At least a bachelor's degree in exercise physiology, nutrition, physical education, or a related field is ideal. In place of formal education, the aspiring personal trainer could seek out informal educational opportunities and document all of the workshops, seminars, conferences, and classes completed. A resume of your education, professional certifications, references, and practical work experience will help you obtain clients.

Second, practical experience is a highly rated qualification. Put yourself in your clients' shoes for a moment. Who would you want to train you, someone with 6 months experience or someone with many years of experience? Students frequently ask: I know I need the experience, but where do I get it? Aspiring personal trainers should seek out local fitness facilities that are willing to let you observe their classes, or even train you. If you have little experience, be willing to serve as an unpaid intern. Anyone who really wants to succeed in this profession needs to be willing to sacrifice and work hard. If your goal is to become a personal trainer, you may need to start at the bottom and work your way up. You know what they say: Just get your foot in the door.

Third, CPR certification is mandatory! CPR classes are offered through hospitals, community centers, and sometimes colleges or universities. A course in basic first aid is also a strong asset.

Fourth, personal trainers should hold a nationally recognized certification. The personal trainer certifications listed in Figure 3.4 have long-standing reputations and appear most frequently in published literature. Which certification should you choose? When someone decides to take a personal training certification, several questions must be considered:

- What are the prerequisites for the exam?
- Do I meet them?
- What do most of the health clubs in my area require?
- What examination do most of the personal trainers I know have?

National Strength and Conditioning Association

Personal trainer	For professionals who train clients in a one-on-one situation in clients' homes, health and fitness clubs, and YMCAs.
Prerequisites	No formal postsecondary coursework or degree is required. Candidates are expected to have a good working knowledge of biomechanical concepts, training adaptations, anatomy, exercise physiology, and program design guidelines.
Certification	120 multiple-choice questions.

Cooper Institute for Aerobics Research

Physical fitness specialist	For individuals who desire training in fitness leadership and the technical skills necessary to implement individualized physical fitness programs.
Prerequisites	Attendance at a 40-hour workshop.
Certification	Exam is written and practical.

American College of Sports Medicine

Health fitness instructor	For candidates who demonstrate competence in exercise fitness testing, designing and executing exercise programs, leading exercise sessions, and operating a fitness facility.
Prerequisites	Bachelor's degree in exercise science, physical education, or allied health.
Certification	Written and practical examination.

American Council on Exercise

Personal trainer	For individuals who work with clients on a one-on-one basis.
Prerequisites	No advanced education is required. Candidates must be 18 years of age and CPR certified.
Certification	Written test only.

Aerobics and Fitness Association of America

Personal trainer–fitness counselor	For fitness professionals who work with clients on a one-on-one basis.
Prerequisites	AFAA primary certification (for aerobics instructors) or successful completion of Introduction to Exercise Science.
Certification	Written and practical examination. Three-day workshop.

Figure 3.4   Personal training certification agencies and requirements.
Adapted from Earnest (1992).

Getting Certified

Becoming a competent personal trainer requires a great deal of skill, knowledge, and experience. It often takes years of hard work and training to become a good personal trainer. Passing a test and "being certified" does not necessarily make you a competent personal trainer! Before attempting to become certified in this speciality, it is recommended that potential candidates take courses in basic and advanced nutrition, exercise physiology, exercise laboratory procedures, fitness design, anatomy and physiology, biomechanics, sports medicine, and weight training. In addition to classroom experience, it is very important to get practical experience.

No amount of knowledge can replace practical experience, especially in the personal training field. Health clubs will often allow you to observe, and sometimes even train you in, a variety of personal training functions. Adequate education, training, and experience are extremely important if you want to become a competent personal trainer.

How much preparation is necessary before attempting to become certified depends on which examination you choose and your current levels of

1. Demonstrate or identify appropriate techniques for health appraisal and use of fitness evaluations.
2. State the purpose and demonstrate basic principles of exercise testing.
3. Describe the categories of participants who should receive medical clearance prior to administration of an exercise test or participation in an exercise program.
4. Identify relative and absolute contraindications to exercise testing or participation.
5. Demonstrate the ability to obtain appropriate medical history, informed consent, and other pertinent information prior to exercise testing.
6. Demonstrate the ability to instruct participants in the use of equipment and test procedures.
7. Demonstrate the ability to assess flexibility, muscular strength, and muscular endurance.
8. Demonstrate various techniques of assessing body composition and discuss the advantages, disadvantages, and limitations of the various techniques.
9. Demonstrate various submaximal and maximal cardiorespiratory-fitness tests using various modes of exercise and interpret the information obtained from the various tests including possible errors.
10. Discuss modification of protocols and procedures for cardiorespiratory-fitness testing in children.
11. Explain the physiological measures that are taken during and after cardiorespiratory-fitness testing.
12. Demonstrate the ability to interpret results of fitness evaluations on apparently healthy individuals and thus with stable disease.
13. Describe and demonstrate techniques for calibration of a cycle ergometer and motor-driven treadmill.
14. Identify appropriate criteria for discontinuing a fitness evaluation and demonstrate proper procedures to be followed after discontinuing such a test.

Figure 3.5 ACSM certification objectives for health appraisal and fitness testing. Reprinted from American College of Sports Medicine (1991).

knowledge and experience. Because individuals who take personal trainer examinations come from such diverse backgrounds, only you can determine the preparation you will need. You must read thoroughly all of the behavioral objectives listed under the examination you decide to take and determine your preparation needs. Figure 3.5 lists the health appraisal and fitness testing behavioral objectives for the American College of Sports Medicine's Health Fitness Instructor Certification.

Use the behavioral objectives listed in Figure 3.5 to help you assess your strengths and weaknesses and to develop a plan of study and practical experience. For some individuals, several weeks is sufficient time to review the material; others may require up to 6 months.

It is important to assess the resources available to help you prepare for a personal training examination. Most health clubs, colleges, and universities offer classes that may be helpful. Practical experience is extremely important for certification. Don't expect to pass a personal training examination if you have only limited practical experience.

Summary

This chapter looked at the qualifications of a personal trainer. Based on national certifications, surveys, and opinions from fitness experts, key qualifications were outlined. This chapter has certainly not identified all of the qualifications needed to be a personal trainer. Attributes such as a friendly and caring personality, desire, and motivation are also important for success as a personal trainer. Certification from a nationally recognized professional organization, documentation of training, education, and experience, will enhance the marketability and respect of personal trainers.

References

American College of Sports Medicine. (1991). *Guidelines for exercise testing and prescription* (4th ed.). Philadelphia: Lea & Febiger.

Brooks, D.S. (1990). *Going solo: The art of personal training*. Los Angeles: Moves International.

Earnest, C. (1992). Personal training: State of the art or state of neglect. *Conditioning Instructor*, **2**(4), 4-11.

National Strength and Conditioning Association (1993). Personal Trainer Certification Registration Brochure. Lincoln, NE: Author.

Thomas, D.Q., Long, K.A., & Myers, B. (1993). Survey of personal trainers in Houston, Texas. *National Strength and Conditioning Association Journal*, **15**(3), 43-46.

Part II
Personal Training as a Business

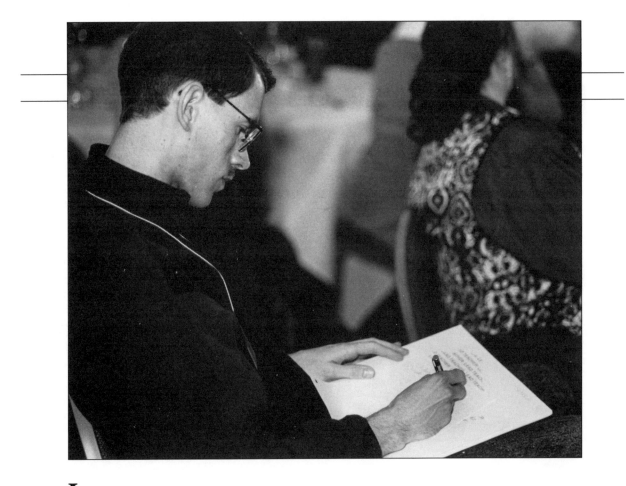

In Part I, personal training was defined, its origin was explored, the qualifications needed to become a personal trainer were discussed, and the fitness industry's view of personal training was presented. The reader should have a good idea of what personal trainers do and where they find employment. In Part II, the business aspects of personal training are presented.

With the exception of people who leave business careers to become personal trainers, or moonlight as personal trainers while holding traditional jobs, most personal trainers do not have any formal education or training in business. Personal trainers learn the business aspects of their trade from experience, by attending conferences and workshops, by reading business journals and books, and by talking with other personal trainers. The primary objective of this book is to present the information new and experienced personal trainers need to become better businesspeople. Some personal trainers have been fortunate enough to have made only a few business mistakes along the way, but there are probably more who have suffered from too many mistakes.

Part II begins with an overview of how to create your own personal training business. In chapter 4, David Rusk, an accountant and personal trainer, shares the knowledge and experience he gained from setting up his own personal training business. One of the first things David talks about is the need to develop a plan and a mission statement. Why do you really want to be a personal trainer? To make money? To help people? Why would someone hire you as a personal trainer? These are questions you need to ask yourself before starting your business. If your goal is to be the best personal trainer in town, or maybe the wealthiest, how are you going to achieve it? You should begin by developing your mission statement. The purpose of developing a mission statement or motto is that it helps you focus on what you want to do best.

In chapter 5, Amy Huggins, a marketing consultant, tells you how to make your company profitable. The best business plan in the world is only as good as the paper it is written on, unless it contains a detailed marketing plan. A good marketing or strategic plan is the essence of successful growth of a company. People often assume that effective marketing takes a great deal of money. In some cases that is true. But there are plenty of stories about executives who developed a great marketing plan, spent millions of dollars to implement it, and were fired because the plan failed! So spending a lot of money on marketing does not guarantee success. There are hundreds of inexpensive and effective ways to market your personal training business, so don't get discouraged if your budget is small.

In chapter 6, Gregory Florez, a successful personal training entrepreneur, shares his wealth of knowledge and experience in setting up a successful personal training company. If your business is started and you have a marketing plan, next you need to manage your business effectively to make it grow. Although managing is probably the least enjoyable part of personal training, it is one of the most essential functions a personal trainer must perform in order to be successful. There are probably just as many personal trainers who leave the business on any given day as there are people entering the fitness business. The reason most leave is lack of business skills.

In chapter 7, David Herbert, a leading legal expert on exercise, teaches you how to reduce the legal risk to your personal training business. Although nobody likes to think about it, the possibility of being sued always exists. By understanding the laws that pertain to personal training and carefully reviewing all aspects of your business, you can reduce the risk of legal problems.

Chapter 4

Creating Your Own Personal Training Business

David B. Rusk

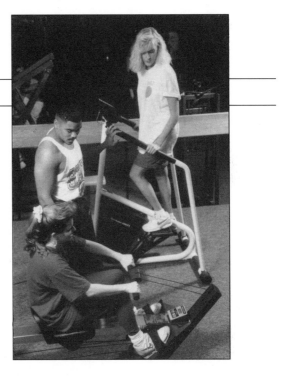

The objectives of this chapter are to

- explain the importance of a mission statement and business plan,
- discuss the pros and cons of sole proprietorship, partnership, and corporation; and
- discuss how to set up and run a personal training business.

Overview

Do you have what it takes to run a business? You know that the experts say that most small businesses fail! Just because you have the desire and expertise to go into business for yourself doesn't mean you will be a success. Each day, thousands of people with a great idea and a lot of determination, often with little or no money, set out to strike it rich. Unfortunately, most of these highly motivated people have little or no idea exactly how they are going to set up and manage their business. Although starting a personal training business or service is not the same as opening a 25,000 sq ft health club, the principles are the same. Any successful businessperson will tell you that you have to have a blueprint or business plan in order to succeed. This chapter presents essential information about starting a personal training business. Even after reading this chapter and the entire book, you should still get advice from an accountant and lawyer before starting a business.

Who would have thought that showing someone how to use free weights and machines at a local gym would evolve into one of the most sought after and lucrative occupations of the 1990s? It was December 1989 that I first read in a major business publication about how personal fitness training would become one of the top 10 occupations of the next decade. You can imagine my excitement; I had just decided to leave accounting and become a personal trainer full time. As I have learned, and those of you reading this book will learn, there is more to personal fitness training than having a degree and being certified. This chapter will address the business aspects of personal training.

Developing a Mission Statement and a Business Plan

Before training starts, before you interview clients, and especially before you accept your first payment, you need to know why you have decided to become a fitness trainer. You need to develop a *mission statement*. A business or corporate mission statement spells out the overall strategy or intent that will govern the goals and objectives of a business or company. Unlike goals, objectives, or both, your mission statement enables you to clarify your purpose for yourself and other interested individuals (e.g., investors, customers, or bankers). A mission statement gives you a direction in order to develop business goals and objectives.

In order to develop a mission statement, you must first state the nature of your business and define the areas of your concentration. For example, a personal trainer might have a mission statement such as:

The mission at ACME Personal Trainers is to provide the highest quality personalized fitness instruction [the nature], using state of the art equipment so our clients can reach all of their fitness and health goals [your areas of concentration].

Your mission statement defines your path, explains your vision, and describes your intentions. As you begin to educate yourself and to add detail to what you will offer to prospective clients, your mission statement will keep you on track. Your mission statement is the foundation from which you will build your business. Below is the NSCA mission statement:

The NSCA, as a nonprofit, worldwide authority on strength and conditioning [the nature] for improved physical performance, creates and disseminates related knowledge and enhances the careers of its members [the area of concentration]. (National Strength and Conditioning Association, 1993)

The NSCA mission statement not only describes what the NSCA is (the nature), but the statement also describes what the NSCA does (the area of concentration). Your mission statement should do the same.

When you get in your car, you usually have a good idea of where you are going and how you are going to get there. When it comes to business, you must have a good idea of where you are going as well. Your *business plan* is your map. Your business plan is proof that you have put some thought into where you want to go and how you will get there. Business plans are not only balance sheets, income statements, and 5-year financial forecasts, business plans also indicate the type of business entity you will be, your company policies, your training rates, your hours of operation, and any other situation that will affect your business.

Choosing a Business Entity

When I started my training business, I had to decide on a business entity. The basic choices are a sole proprietorship, a partnership, or a corporation. As indicated below, each has its own advantages and disadvantages. Your choice should be reflective of your personality and your vision as stated in the mission statement mentioned earlier.

Sole Proprietorship

A sole-proprietorship business is owned and operated by one individual. I decided on a sole proprietorship because I wanted ease in making decisions and running the business. Although a sole proprietorship has the lowest start-up costs, is easy to form, has no division of profits, and has no one else in the decision-making process, there are some disadvantages. A sole proprietor assumes responsibility for all decisions, good or bad, is personally liable for all business debts, and has trouble raising capital for future business expansion. When there is a problem, the sole proprietor is the only one who can deal with it!

In addition, a sole proprietor needs to obtain a business license in the jurisdiction where the business is located. When a sole proprietor operates a business in a name other than his or her own, notice must be given to the business community in the form of a DBA or "doing business as" ad printed in the local newspaper. This procedure, in addition to letting the community know who you are, also serves as a name search performed by the paper to make sure no one else is using your business name.

Partnership

A business partnership is defined as a business owned and operated by two or more people. I never considered a partnership, but there are some advantages to this form of business. The start-up costs are moderately low, there is ease in formation, more than one person is involved in the decision-making process, and because of your partners' added assets, more capital is available. The biggest obstacle in forming a partnership is finding an honest, compatible partner; many partnerships fail because of partner fraud or incompatibility. Also, the partners are liable for partnership debts, and there is a division of profits. Before going into a business with someone, make sure you know all you can about that person; also, have an attorney prepare a contract that outlines each partner's roles and responsibilities.

The advantages of partnerships and sole proprietorships include

- ease of formation,
- low cost of formation,
- ability to operate in different states without registration,
- exemption from business taxes (only owners pay taxes), and
- minimal government regulation (American Council on Exercise, 1991).

Corporation

A corporation is defined as a business that operates as an independent legal entity, separate from the owners. One of the benefits of incorporating is protecting personal assets, but incorporating is expensive, must follow many legal regulations, and slows down the ability to make important decisions. Each of us has to decide what type of entity is best; but remember, we are professionals, we are legitimate, and must satisfy all relevant government regulations. Setting up a corporation is an expensive and complicated task; be sure to get good legal and tax advice before setting up a corporation.

The disadvantages of corporations include

- complicated legal requirements,
- high costs of formation,
- registration requirements in each state where business is conducted,
- taxation on both the owners and the corporation, and
- extensive government regulation (American Council on Exercise, 1991).

Setting Business Policies

So, you've decided on a business entity; now you must decide how you will run your business. A number of business policies must be formulated. Each client must be made aware of your cancellation, no-show, and late policies. It is not uncommon for a trainer to require a 24-hour notice of cancellation in order for the client not to be charged for a workout session. After all, trainers arrange their daily schedules based on client appointments. Trainers need to keep their schedules filled. Obviously, someone not showing up for a scheduled workout should still be charged for that hour. In addition, clients need to know what to expect if they are late for an appointment. I charge for sessions in which the client is late 15 minutes or more. Remember, you are a professional and this is your business. See Figure 4.1 for an example of a personal trainer's policies and procedures.

How will your clients pay for their sessions? Will you bill them or will you ask them to prepay? There are trainers who use both methods. I prefer to have my clients prepay for their sessions, because this enhances their commitment. In addition, should a problem arise over payment for a missed session or late arrival, it is much easier to keep your fee if you already have the client's money than to bill for a disputed session. I let my clients know they must make another payment 1 week before the payment is actually due. This allows them to bring their next payment at the time of the last paid session. Be careful about clients who make a habit of forgetting their checks. These clients need to be reminded that you are a professional and that you expect to be treated like one. If you decide to bill your clients at the end of each month, be sure to itemize all charges, including those charges for missed and late sessions.

The length of your training session and its components should be explained to each client. Most training sessions last 1 hour and include a warm-up, workout, and cool-down. The warm-up and cool-down can be done without the trainer after these program components have been explained to the client. Remember, however, the trainer should tailor the workout session to meet the needs, goals, and capabilities of the client.

Clients need to feel comfortable when they are working out; however, they should also wear clothes appropriate for the environmental conditions. Shortly

---

Each training session is based on a 60-minute workout. To get the most out of our efforts, please be ready to exercise at the appointed time.

If you are more than 15 minutes late for a scheduled session, it will be considered a no-show and you will be charged.

As a professional courtesy, there will be no charge on sessions that are canceled with a 24-hour notice.

Always pay for your session in advance. This will reserve a scheduled time and help you commit to your goals.

Cash payments are preferred, but personal checks are accepted. If a check is returned (NSF), cash will be required for all future payments.
Payments will be made _____ .

Session payments are nonrefundable, but they may be transferred. Unused sessions must be used within 30 days of the last completed session.

As a courtesy, please give a 14-day notice prior to terminating services.

The first session consists of your initial fitness profile and the purchase of the nutrition handbook.

Please wear loose, comfortable clothing to facilitate ease of movement, along with appropriate athletic footwear, and weight lifting gloves when needed. Always bring a towel and water bottle to sessions.

Business hours are 7:00 a.m. - 6:00 p.m.

Thank you!

By signing here, I agree to the program and payment policy.

Name _____   Date _____

Figure 4.1   Sample program and payment policy.

---

after I started my training business, I had T-shirts printed with my logo on them. I gave one to each of my clients. Not only did this give the client something to wear at the gym, but it was also great advertising.

Session Rates

One of the most difficult decisions I had to make when starting out was what to charge for my training sessions. Should I give discounts to customers who, for example, offered to pay cash or who agreed to pay for 3 months in advance? I attended personal training seminars and read many articles addressing this issue. Each time the answer was the same. Decide on an hourly rate or a fee schedule and stick to it, no matter what. I never realized how many deal-makers there were until I started personal training.

The first step in the process of determining what your rates will be is to find what other trainers in your geographical area charge. For example, the rates that I charge in Long Beach, California, are quite different from the rates charged by trainers in Beverly Hills and Hollywood. Examine the economic health of

your region and get an understanding of what your market will bear. Another very important point to consider when setting your rates is your level of expertise and experience. Obviously, someone with a bachelor's degree, right out of school, would not charge as much as someone with a master's degree who has 10 years of training experience.

Business Records

Personal fitness training is a business and, as such, record keeping is essential. Records showing business income and all business-related expenses must be maintained. Third parties, such as your bankers (when you request a loan for expansion or buying new equipment) and your accountant (to prepare your tax returns), need your business records. You need records to compare actual figures to your budgeted figures. Most of us have calculated how much money we need in order to pay our bills. When starting a business, these calculations are a very important part of the business plan. If actual figures do not match budgeted figures, then changes can be made to get your business on the right track. Part of the record-keeping work is keeping track of client sessions. I use a daily planner to schedule workout times and any other events that I need to remember (see Figure 4.2). I keep a workout card for each client; the cards list session dates and record the exercises performed. If a client cancels a session, I note the reason. I also note whether the client was charged or not, and why. These workout cards have come in handy several times when I have needed to reconcile payments and sessions with clients.

Introductory Documentation

You have written your mission statement and business plan, decided on a business entity, and determined company policies and session rates. You must now consider documents that you will use to introduce yourself and your services to prospective clients, get information about your clients, and obtain personal liability documents.

Creating a Presentation Package

In 1986, as a trainer new to the business, I needed a way to introduce myself to prospective clients. I wanted my presentation package to provide information about my background and about my training philosophy and training methods. Most prospective clients want to know about the trainer's education, so I decided to create a resume that included my education and experience (see Figure 4.3). I also included a short biography. In addition to providing a resume and short biography, I also wanted to list the components of my program. Your program components will be a mirror of your training philosophies. An example of your training components is how you incorporate strength training, cardiovascular exercise, and flexibility workouts into your sessions. Is nutrition guidance a part of your program? If so, tell your prospective clients what they will learn and what their responsibilities will be.

For example, I have clients keep a daily record of the foods they eat. In addition, they record the times the foods were eaten and any special circumstances like being at a party or just being stressed out for some reason. Because of the question of ethics (we are not registered dietitians or licensed nutritionists)

I do not create a specific menu for my clients. What we are able to do, however, is create an awareness of what is being eaten as well as teach general nutrition facts upon which each client can draw when making food choices.

Personal Liability Documents

The client has reviewed your presentation package and has decided to hire you. At this point your clients must complete information-gathering forms and personal liability documents. Information-gathering documents will help you design appropriate exercise routines. These documents ask about medical histories, lifestyles, exercise, and nutrition habits. All trainers need to know as much as possible about their clients. Would you want to train a client who has diabetes or has suffered a recent heart attack without first knowing about these conditions? I cannot stress enough the importance of obtaining as much information about your client as possible! My medical, lifestyle, and exercise questionnaire is seven pages long and includes questions about the client's eating, drinking, and smoking habits. Make sure your questionnaire is easy to complete and that you obtain the necessary health-related information.

We live in an era where the courts are filled with professional malpractice lawsuits. As part of my document package, I include an informed consent and a waiver of liability. An informed consent basically states that the client knows what the training consists of, as explained in the program components, and is physically capable of performing the required tasks. The waiver of liability releases the trainer from responsibility when the client errs. You must understand that trainer negligence is not protected under any document. For further protection you need to be covered by professional liability insurance. Contact your professional training organization for professional liability insurance information.

Finally, I suggest you hire a professional designer to create your business logo. Your business logo is your most important asset, other than your training talents. It will be your informal introduction to most business relationships. When I started training in 1986, one of the first things I did was to have a logo designed. My thinking was that over time, people would associate my logo with quality personal training and with my name. When you see the golden arches you immediately think of McDonald's and their hamburgers; when people see my logo they immediately think of David Rusk and personal training!

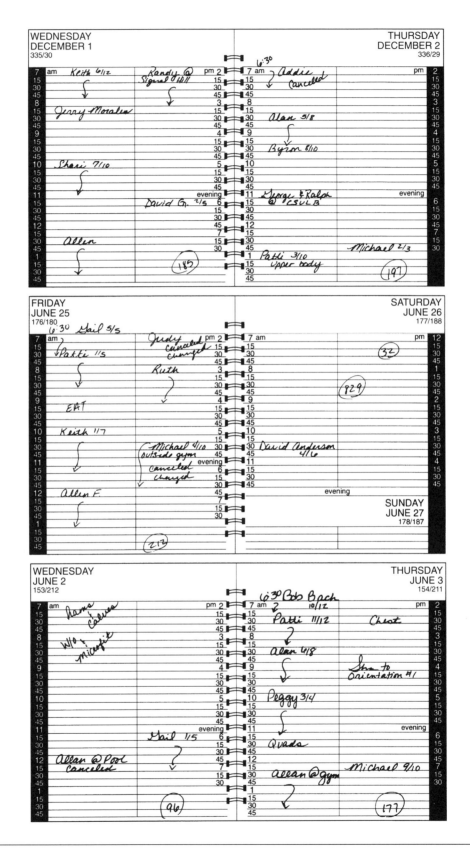

Figure 4.2 Sample daily log.

David Rusk
Certified Strength and Conditioning Specialist
P.O. Box 3522
Long Beach, CA 90803

Objective	To acquire an ever-increasing level of knowledge to draw upon when working with those who seek a higher level of wellness.
Education	
1972-1977	University of Cincinnati, Cincinnati, Ohio Bachelor of Business Administration Major in Accounting
Certificates	
1991	University of California at Irvine Certificate in Fitness Instruction
1989	American College of Sports Medicine Health Fitness Instructor
1987	National Strength and Conditioning Association Certified Stength and Conditioning Specialist
Experience	
1993	Gold's Gym, Long Beach, California Assistant Head Trainer Owner of Microfit, Computerized Fitness Assessment
1989-1992	The Belmont Racquetball and Fitness Club Personal Training Coordinator Restructured a failing program into a successful program
1986-1989	Family Fitness Center, Lakewood, California Developed and operated a personal training program
Achievements	
1993-1994	Speaker at the 1993 and 1994 NSCA National Conferences Commissioned by the NSCA to author a chapter in a book on personal training Second place in a natural bodybuilding contest
Personal Data	Married, one child

• **Fitness and nutrition consultant** • **Personal trainer** •

Figure 4.3   Sample personal training resume.

Summary

Going into business for yourself requires a great deal of planning. Whatever you do, don't rush into it! Take your time and prepare your business plan, mission statement, and client presentation folder. It is wise to consult with an attorney and tax expert before going into business. Professional advice is expensive, but you can't afford not to get it! Talk with other personal trainers who have gone into business for themselves, find out what worked for them and what did not. The best advice you'll get when contemplating going into business for yourself is to try and learn from other people's mistakes.

References

American Council on Exercise. (1991). *Personal Training Manual.* San Diego, CA: Author.

National Strength and Conditioning Association. (April 1993). *NSCA Mission Statement.* Strategic Planning Workgroup (1994) Revised By-Laws.

Chapter 5

Marketing Your Personal Training Business

Amy T. Huggins

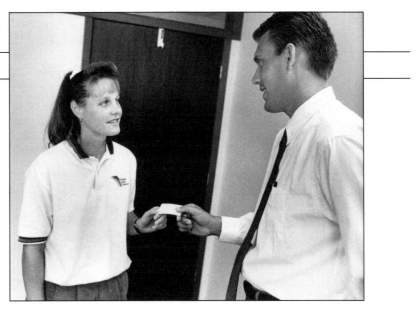

The objectives of this chapter are to

- define basic marketing terms,
- develop a marketing plan,
- determine the price of your services,
- review marketing plan tools, and
- discuss selling strategies.

Overview

O.K., so you did it! You went into business for yourself. Why aren't people knocking on your door for your services? The next step in operating a successful business is to learn about marketing. It may happen in the movies, but just because you built it, that doesn't mean they will come! Chapter 5 presents essential information on how to market your personal training business. Marketing is often overlooked when setting up a small business. It is possible to spend too much time and money on marketing and get very little in return for your investment. This chapter introduces basic marketing principles. You will learn how to develop a marketing plan and how to sell your services. If you want to be a financially successful personal trainer, you need to become good at marketing your business!

You are a professional, a personal trainer who seeks to become knowledgeable and competent before training others. Most people interested in the field of personal training prepare themselves with thorough training in the physical realm; they study, for example, exercise physiology, nutrition, stretching, and strength training. Yet this book claims that regardless of how much training you receive in these physical areas, success will elude you until you are also schooled in the business of personal training.

One of the most important aspects of running a business is marketing. Think a moment—do you know any business or profession that does not market itself? Some businesses are more discreet in their marketing efforts than screaming cable TV advertisers, but even doctors, lawyers, and presidents market themselves. This is not to say that you haven't already marketed yourself or another company's products or services successfully. In fact, some reflection on your past marketing successes will help you decide where you can best devote your time and money in the future. The most effective marketing efforts will be substantially enhanced if you have a plan.

To begin, it is important to develop a traditional strategic marketing plan. But given the highly competitive nature of the economy and the fragmented structure of the personal training industry, you will also want to study the section on developing a creative marketing plan. The reason why a traditional plan is not sufficient is deeper than the nature of the economy and the structure of an industry; highly successful companies are enormously creative with their marketing and reap enormous returns on their marketing investments. Read on.

Develop a Traditional Strategic Marketing Plan

The key components of a strategic marketing plan are the five *P*s:

1. Product (or service)
2. Pricing
3. Place (or location)
4. People
5. Positioning

The five *P*s are the fundamental building blocks of a strategic marketing plan. In other words, they are a useful way of organizing your thoughts about what you are going to do, where you will do it, how you will price it, who you want to work with, and how you will talk about your product or service.

Whether you are beginning a new personal training business or you are a seasoned professional ready to move to the next stage in your career, spend the time to think, dream, and clarify your answers to these questions. Let's look at each *P* in more detail.

Offer a Product or Service

You may think this is obvious—you are offering the service of personal training. Because you are selling this service, you need to be specific about its components so you can give clear answers to questions from prospective clients.

For example, what does your training qualify you to offer? What kind of training will your personal training session typically include? How long will each session be? What service standards will you establish regarding professionalism, dependability, safety, and quality? Finally the most important question: How is your service distinct? What is your competitive edge?

Develop a Specialty

One way to differentiate your service is to offer a unique type of training by specializing, for example, in strength training or in conditioning for a specific sport, like skiing or golf. Another way trainers identify themselves is by serving a special population, such as people with a medical condition (e.g., diabetics or arthritic patients), people in a clearly definable population (e.g., seniors), or people in a specific profession (e.g., airline pilots or lawyers).

Whatever you choose as a specialty, be sure that you do so because you have a passion for it. This element of passion is crucial because you must thirst for the knowledge it takes to develop the specialty and because it will be natural for you to market it to clients and referral sources.

As Adrienne Jamiel indicated in her article, "The Specialist's Strategy to Build a Client Base" (Jamiel, 1993), there are several steps to take to find your passion and determine the endeavor you truly want to pursue. (Use Figure 5.1 to help you find your passion.) In Step 1, quickly write all your thoughts about what you dream you can do; then choose two areas that hold interest and promise for you. To determine the feasibility of these two ideas, Step 2 is to talk with people who are currently working in the area you want to pursue about the challenges and rewards of this line of work and to research the topics via seminars, lectures, and library resources.

Step 3 in this process is to experiment. If you want to give a mind–body movement class, offer it to a

The first step in finding your passion is to list all thoughts that have ever occurred to you about what you would like to do as a personal trainer. Be patient and tremendously creative as you list at least 20 ideas. (See examples below.) Then narrow your choices to two ideas. Realize that what you choose could also differentiate your services from other trainers' and thereby become your competitive edge over them.

1. _____   (example: work with senior citizens)
2. _____   (example: work with new mothers)
3. _____   (example: work with top executives at Microsoft)
4. _____
5. _____
6. _____
7. _____
8. _____
9. _____
10. _____
11. _____
12. _____
13. _____
14. _____
15. _____
16. _____
17. _____
18. _____
19. _____
20. _____

Figure 5.1   Finding-your-passion worksheet.

group of friends or sit in on another related class and offer to help the instructor. The idea is to perform your dream.

Then you must evaluate. After researching and performing your dream, Step 4 is to decide if this idea is still as interesting as you originally thought; whether you have the necessary expertise to continue, or know where to get it; and if your dream is marketable in your community. A mind–body movement class, for example, would be more successful in a resort community or a large city than in a small town.

The last steps, 5, 6, and 7, encourage you to envision your future doing this specialty, to declare your commitment to it, and market it—to clients, other trainers, allied health professionals, and charities. The author concludes that "when you build your

client base around a specialty that you're passionate about and put out the word that you have something of value to share, rest assured—your clients will find you" (Jamiel, 1993).

Consider Offering Products

Although they are primarily selling a service, many trainers improve their income potential by also offering products. There are literally hundreds of types of products you could offer, but if you choose to sell products to your clients, be sure that the ones you choose to represent are consistent with the standards you set for the type of training you provide and the needs of your clients.

For example, many clients will turn to you for advice on nutritional products. Although some products, like dietary supplements or reducers, may be easy to sell and quite profitable, what image do these products lend to the professional quality of your training service? In addition, some manufacturers require that you become a distributor and maintain an inventory of products, which may tie up your money and become a burden to sell. There are some excellent computerized nutritional analysis tools available, yet these require an up-front investment for the computer hardware, software, and training. Carefully research all products you want to sell. How does the quality of these products compare to similar ones? Is the pricing competitive with similar products? If you have to become a distributor, how large is the investment? Do you have to carry inventory? Does the manufacturer provide product and sales training? How long has the company been in business?

A simple way to meet your clients' need for nutritional education is to offer another service, such as a grocery store tour where you teach clients how to choose healthier foods where they normally shop. And, of course, you can always refer your client to a qualified dietitian.

Establish Pricing Practices

This area includes not only product or service pricing, but your payment policy.

Pricing for your personal training services should be based on

- your costs,
- your profit margin,
- your competition, and
- your market.

Your costs fall into two categories: variable and fixed. Fixed costs stay the same month-to-month or year-to-year; fixed costs include rent and personal liability insurance. Variable costs change frequently and depend upon how your business is structured. If you train clients in their homes, variable costs include the clothing you wear for work, your utility and phone charges, your business cards and stationery, the training equipment you purchase, and the costs of gasoline, car maintenance, and insurance. If you train clients in a facility, your variable costs will include clothing, business cards, and self-promotion. Or if you have other trainers working for you, payroll is also a variable cost. Up to 80% of what you charge for personal training should cover the variable and fixed costs of your business.

Next, include your profit margin in your pricing as a fixed item, nonnegotiable, because you need to pay yourself and save for unpredicted expenses. It

can vary from 10% to 40% of your price, but is also determined by the market forces of competition and the demographics of the market you serve.

Your pricing should be competitive with what the other trainers in your market are charging. If you offer a specialized service for physical rehab patients, you may be able to charge a premium between 5% to 10%. But be aware of what your competitors are charging because your clients will know and ask you about it.

Finally, your pricing should be sensitive to the socioeconomic status of the market you serve. Because of the lesser number of high-wage earners in Kenosha, Wisconsin, versus the number in a city like Chicago, for example, a trainer in Kenosha would be wise to offer a discounted price.

So let's look at an example of how to establish a price. Suppose some of your clients asked for a well-planned nutritional program that was easy to follow. You research the field and decide to sell a program called Think Lite. The fixed cost of the product was based on the quantity you ordered, but because you only wanted five kits, your unit cost was $35. The total shipping charge was $4.82, making your total cost per unit almost $36. No one else in your area sells Think Lite, but the kits are selling for $50 to $80 elsewhere. Competing diet programs in your region have low introductory costs, but the total program cost is usually in the hundreds of dollars for special food and material purchases. You decide to sell the kits for $49.95, plus tax, earning a nice profit of $14 per kit (nearly 40%) because the below-$50 price compares favorably with other local dietary programs and is in line with the local economy.

Finally, pricing also requires that you make some decisions about how you will be paid for your products and services. Most people prefer to be billed for their purchases, so you need an accounting system for invoicing customers and receiving payments. Many trainers bill their clients in advance so that the client has monetary commitment to come to each session and so that if the client cancels too late or misses an appointment, the trainer is still compensated. Will you accept cash? Checks? Credit cards? What will be your payment terms, for example, payable within 15 days of receipt? Payable immediately? What will you do if clients don't pay? All of these questions, and your answers, are part of your strategic marketing plan.

Select a Place or Location

As a personal trainer, there are many places you can work: in clients' homes, in a studio or health club, in an apartment or condominium exercise facility, or in a public YMCA or corporate facility. Many trainers actually work in a variety of places, recognizing that each offers different opportunities for attracting and serving clients.

For example, if you live in a large metropolitan area, unique opportunities exist. The new apartment complex has an outdoor pool, so you offer personalized aqua training sessions for parents, children, and visiting grandparents. If a local corporation does not have a health facility, but incurs substantial health-care costs, you can lead a walking club to help reduce on-the-job stress and blood pressure (Rippe & Ward, 1989). If both the apartment and corporate facilities have unused rooms, you can become their consultant and trainer and help choose appropriate exercise equipment and lead fitness sessions for residents or employees.

Oh, but you live in a smaller town. Then check whether the local YMCA or health club needs personal training. Check with the park district about leading walks through one of the attractive parks. What about the local fire fighters, police department, and nurses and nurse assistants who must use their backs to lift and carry elderly patients? Are these people in good enough physical condition to do their jobs without injuring themselves?

Use your imagination and consider the local opportunities for business development in your strategic marketing plan.

Target a Group of People

This *P* refers not to who you'll work for, or who will work with you, but who will buy what you have to sell.

The demographics of any group are identified by their age, sex, race, socioeconomic level, and education. So you may determine that your best clients are females, aged 30 to 55, of any race, who have at least a college degree, and earn over $25,000 annually. You may want to define them even more by life situation, for example, women who have had children or who work full time; or by psychographics, for example, women who are interested in self-improvement; or by where they live.

The advantage of determining the demographics and psychographics of the population you plan to serve is that it focuses your marketing efforts on a particular *target market*. The more you can focus on your target market, the more you will benefit from the best marketing tool available, word-of-mouth. The caution about focusing exclusively on one target is that you may develop tunnel vision and consider

only 30-year-old professionals, ignoring the needs of a 26-year-old manicurist who is very interested in your work.

In addition, the more that you can differentiate your target from the competition, the better. One successful personal trainer targets adults who ski competitively, which is clearly a very closely defined target. This type of targeting develops a niche, and thus a competitive edge, for your training business.

Position Your Business

The final *P* is positioning, or the way you choose to identify your business. A business positions itself with a name and a short phrase describing its business. A public radio station, for example, named KUOW in Seattle, follows its call letters with the slogan "Bringing You the World." Some business names are very descriptive, like "Salsaerobics, Inc." or "Body Business, Inc." The name I chose for my personal training business is "Well Beings, Inc." because I wanted to communicate that whether we trained individuals, spoke at a convention, or delivered a seminar for a corporation, our work was to improve well-being.

If you are beginning your own personal training business, no doubt you are anxious to develop a name. But remember that whatever name you choose, it must serve you for the long term, while you build your reputation and your business. Will the name keep on working for you even if your business changes so you are doing a different kind of training or change your focus? Will you still like the name 5 years from now? If your name includes your geographical area, what will happen if you move?

I ask these questions because all these things happened to Well Beings and me. My business changed when I became a mother, because I could train people only when I could find daycare. So rather than working during early morning, later evening, and weekend hours, I trained during daytime. To supplement my reduced income, I increased my marketing to corporations for in-house training on healthier employee lifestyles. After 5 years, I like the name Well Beings, Inc., even more!

Survey the names of personal training businesses in your market area. How are other personal training, massage, and nutrition services named? If you are the only trainer in a small town, maybe you want to name your business Ashland Personal Training, for example, to represent the local focus you're providing. Other trainers use their name, such as O'Grady Fitness, Inc. But the larger your market, the more you should seek to develop a business name that has broad and long-range applicability.

How do you develop a name? Think creatively and wildly. Ask everyone you meet, and brainstorm with your friends and family. Figure 5.2 will help you generate as many ideas as possible (at least 20); narrow down your choice to one or two names. Go back to the same people who helped you generate names and ask them to choose between the two you like best. The more you talk about it, the more comfortable you will become with your choice.

The next step is to get business cards and stationery. You can probably design and print the template of what you want on a computer, or find a friend or small business that provides a design service. Then go to any local print shop to choose paper and colors and order a quantity of business cards and letterhead stationery.

It is important to take these steps because, as discussed later, selling personal training is difficult. It is an intangible product, and having a business name, business cards, and stationery all create tangibility that reinforces the quality you represent and what you provide. Your printed materials will be the tools you use throughout the implementation of your marketing plan.

The reason to develop a marketing plan is so that your efforts to promote yourself are not wasted. That means that the efforts support one another, for example, an article you wrote appears in the section of the newspaper where you also advertise; and that your marketing is cost effective, for example, that

---

Brainstorm!! Ask your friends and family, people you know in business, or complete strangers to help you name your personal training business. Tell them what you want to do as a personal trainer; that may help them and you think of an appropriate name. Be patient and tremendously creative as you list at least 20 ideas. (See examples below.) Then narrow your choices to your two favorites and ask your helpers to choose one.

1. _____ (example: Ski Energy)
2. _____ (example: Body Power, Inc.)
3. _____ (example: Flex-Appeal Training)
4. _____
5. _____
6. _____
7. _____
8. _____
9. _____
10. _____
11. _____
12. _____
13. _____
14. _____
15. _____
16. _____
17. _____
18. _____
19. _____
20. _____

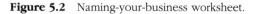

Figure 5.2   Naming-your-business worksheet.

you receive a discounted ad rate because you run your ad multiple times.

The preliminary step toward establishing a marketing plan is to develop a marketing schedule and budget. Ideally, you want to promote yourself continuously, a task that is difficult to manage as your training hours become booked. So your marketing plan must be developed with a sensitivity to the time it takes to do a task, as well as its cost. For example, you may choose public speaking as one of your marketing efforts, but if you are not a competent speaker, you may invest more time and money in learning to speak well, writing, and delivering your speech than you receive in client revenues.

The final thing to be aware of before you actually design your marketing plan is the issue of intangibility. People buy a car, perfume, food, or any other product partially on the basis of information, but they largely rely on their senses—how it looks, sounds, feels, tastes, smells. Personal training is a service that can promise future results but doesn't have anything for the prospect to see or hold. However, you can offer a tangible "taste" of your services. Offer clients a shortened training session or show them a program you designed for another client. Show the client before and after pictures of another client and provide phone references. Invite prospects to one of your public talks or to join a grocery shopping tour where you teach another client how to choose lowfat, nutritious foods. Whatever you do, let prospects touch, feel, see, or hear the benefits of personal training.

To assist you in developing your own five Ps, your product or service, pricing, positioning, place, and people, please take time to work on Figure 5.3. Then you'll be ready to choose the tools you'll use for your marketing plan.

Plan Your Marketing Tools

There are at least nine effective ways for companies to promote themselves and their products to their target market.

1. *Referrals:* both to and from related health professionals (e.g., a physical therapist)
2. *Direct marketing:* any printed material mailed to a target group
3. *Advertising:* traditional paid media advertising (e.g., newspaper, local radio)
4. *Public speaking:* sharing your knowledge with the public (you usually get paid)
5. *Networking:* attending meetings, phoning associates to provide supportive information, referring clients

6. *Publicity:* print or radio information about you or your business (free)
7. *Donation:* you donate your services to a charity (a type of publicity)
8. *Word-of-mouth:* recommendation (or not) from a client or referer to a prospect (can be good or bad)
9. *Telemarketing:* selling services over the phone to strangers

Within each of these categories, there are many variations. For example, you can also advertise in magazines, on cable TV, on network TV, in an association newsletter, or on a bus. Before you choose any marketing vehicle, advertising, or direct mail, you need to ask two questions: (a) Does it reach your target effectively? and (b) What is the cost per prospect reached?

These are key questions. For instance, you may be honored to speak at the local Jaycees meeting, but it may be attended only by working men, and your target is women. On the other hand, you'll want to do some things just to build awareness of your business and what you provide. Nevertheless, don't get caught thinking you are building awareness if you find yourself always donating your services, speaking for free, and making unpaid appearances. You are in business and deserve to be paid!

Key Issues: Time and Money

So which marketing tools will you choose? Depending upon your budget, who can be reached most cost effectively, and how much time you regularly plan to devote to marketing, choose at least five methods. Why five? Because even if you choose commercial TV because of its wide reach, your prospect may not watch anything but public TV. However, if you also write an article for the association she belongs to, give a brown-bag lunch speech on executive fitness at her company, exchange business cards with her at a networking meeting, and get referred to her by her massage therapist, she will hear enough about you to move her from just being aware of your business to being interested in paying for your services.

Finally, take all your marketing methods and schedule them, trying to do at least one thing every month. If you think that after the winter holidays is a promising time to generate new business, then plan to reserve some time in October, November, and December to plan your marketing campaign.

For example, let's say you wanted to (a) send out a promotional postcard (direct mail) to a carefully identified list, (b) be interviewed on a radio show, and

Use the space below to develop your five *P*s.

1. Product or Service

The product(s) I plan to offer (include description of type of training, service standards, duration of each training session, competitive edge [specialty] for each product):

1.
2.
3.

The service(s) I will offer:

2. Pricing

The amount I charge for each product and service listed above, considering variable and fixed costs and my profit margin:

My billing terms and policy:

Will I charge clients who cancel or miss appointments?

What forms of payment will I accept?

3. Place

I will provide my services at the following locations:

4. People

The target market for my products and services is (include description by age, sex, income, marital status, education, life situation, and psychographics):

5. Positioning

My business name is (from Figure 5.2):

My competitive edge (passion) is (from Figure 5.1):

How will I answer the question, "What do you do?"

Figure 5.3   Worksheet for the 5 *P*s of your strategic marketing plan.

(c) make a presentation at a professional-women's networking group. In early October, you get a list of the professional-women's groups in your area and begin calling their program coordinators with an offer to speak at their January meetings. The title of your speech is "How to Exercise Safely and Effectively in the Winter." You also find out which local radio stations do interviews and begin calling station managers to establish contacts and make your offer. Finally, you begin work on the promotional postcard and compile a mailing list that hits your target.

Notice how November and December are filled with following-through activities—designing and printing the postcard, printing mailing labels, and finally, timing the mailing so your cards won't be lost in Christmas mail. You also need time for booking a presentation, sending the organization a biography and speech outline for its internal publicity promotion to their members, and preparing the presentation. Don't forget about scheduling the interview, calling to confirm it, and arriving early. Marketing effectively takes time and energy, and some money, but the return on your investment in January and beyond can be substantial.

Depending upon the quality of your mailing list, it's possible that 10% to 12% of your direct mail recipients will respond favorably to your mailing. If you send 200 postcards, you could generate 20 to 24 qualified leads. At your presentation, out of 45 people attending, 10 to 15 ask for more information. And you received 20 phone calls after the radio interviewer mentioned the name of your business several times. Out of the 60 qualified leads you generated in January, you have 15 new clients! What a profitable New Year's gift to yourself!

Always Promote Yourself

Obviously, not all months are going to be as filled with marketing activities as the 4-month period just described, but as I already recommended, you should promote yourself constantly. How? By asking and by observing.

Ask your clients, other health professionals, and friends for referrals. "You know, I build my business through many different marketing efforts. But by far, the most cost-effective and personal method is through referrals and word-of-mouth. Would you be willing to recommend my services to others? To follow through, I would call the person, introduce myself, and offer a free sample [e.g., training session] of what I provide."

Observation is another excellent way to boost your business. When I attended my first personal training convention with IDEA, the association of fitness professionals, I heard Anne Kashiwa, then the national spokesperson for the Rockport Company, mention her son as she led several sessions on fitness walking. After her presentation, I introduced myself and asked how she managed traveling on business for Rockport and the responsibilities of motherhood. She indicated that traveling nationwide was difficult. I suggested that as the national spokesperson, she could recommend that Rockport hire regional representatives partly to reduce her travel burden. A year later, Rockport announced the Rockport Ambassador program and hired and trained nine representatives around the country—including me. I observed a need and created an opportunity.

Well, you may think, I can't ask people to refer me or suggest that a company create a regional spokesperson network. Yes you can. Success requires optimism, interpersonal communication skills, creativity, and resourcefulness. This may sound like a demanding list, but these are skills you can develop.

In *Learned Optimism*, Martin Seligman (Seligman, 1991) describes his research on animals and humans that shows conclusively that what he calls our "explanatory style" greatly influences our abilities and our health. Included in the book is a questionnaire to help readers determine if they are more likely to explain phenomena in an optimistic or pessimistic way. Seligman applied his theories to the sales and promotion efforts of life insurance salespeople and found that those who were optimistic persevered in the face of rejection, while those who were pessimistic gave up. I recommend this book so you can discover your own explanatory style, and if you choose, take actions to modify it, and so you can more easily understand your clients' reactions to certain events. This book addresses two important business requirements: optimism and interpersonal communication skills.

Beth Rothenberg, owner of Sidekicks Personal Training and coauthor of *Touch Training for Strength* (Rothenberg & Rothenberg, 1994), is the most resourceful and creative personal trainer I've ever met. And she is successful partly because of these skills. You forgot your free weights? Use one of your client's tables to do isometric leg presses, triceps dips, and push-ups. Out of Dynabands or rubber bands? Use a towel and your own body to provide resistance for adductor and abductor exercises. Didn't remember the step bench today? Use the stairs and an ironing board for reverse curl and gravity-resistant sit-ups. Grab the kid's ball and use it between the client's legs for sit-ups, inner thigh work, and calf raises. The list goes on and on, depending upon your creativity and resourcefulness.

What do these skills have to do with marketing? Everything! The client who sees your resourcefulness and creativity will be happy to refer you to friends and tell others about your creative training methods. Doctors and physical therapists with demanding schedules will gladly refer clients who need a good listener to you. The personal trainer who is optimistic and creative will always keep selling rather than give up.

Practice Good Selling Skills

The final phase of marketing, once you have developed your target and actually obtained a lead for a qualified prospect, is to close the sale. You begin by contacting prospects on the phone. To avoid playing phone tag, you may want to call after regular work hours or on weekends. Briefly explain how you obtained that person's name and the services you offer. Ask about their concerns in the areas of fitness and nutrition. Then listen, ask questions, and listen some more to learn as much as possible about your prospects.

Finally, make an offer. "It sounds to me like you're concerned because you have gained weight since you quit smoking and have not been able to take it off. Is that accurate? I'd like to continue this conversation with you in person, so I can understand more about your attempts to lose weight and do a health assessment that will help us work together. I don't charge for this assessment, and it is a good opportunity for us to become acquainted. Is 9:00 a.m. or 1:00 p.m. better for you on Saturday?"

On Saturday, arrive promptly and dress professionally. Remember, the first 3 to 5 minutes are the key moments to express your confidence, professionalism, and interest. Reiterate what you discussed on the phone, and ask more questions about the prospect's health history. (You should have a health screening form, as described in chapter 6.) Then allow your prospect to ask any questions about your service and how you would address specific concerns. Present yourself as a partner dedicated to solving your prospect's problem.

The next step is to ask prospects what standards or goals must be met for them to be satisfied. This is a very useful discussion because it is important for you to understand the client's expectations. For instance, if your client has a friend or associate who has a personal trainer, then your client may have preconceived ideas about the amount of time it will take to reach a special goal or about "extras" the trainer provides, like informational articles. Even if your client doesn't have specific ideas about your

relationship, this is a good time to explain how you work with a client and see if this prospect would want or need anything else.

Finally, you can outline your policies regarding payment, cancellations, and refunds. Then to close the sale, ask for it. At Well Beings, we asked for the sale by having a fill-in-the-blank contract that stated who would be working with the client, how frequently, at what times, the number of sessions, and the cost to the client. It also detailed our policy on cancellation and liability and listed the goals the client wanted to achieve with our help. After completing the form, the trainer and the client would sign it; that act closed the sale.

If you have a prospect who is uncomfortable filling out the form after your discussion, you may need to offer your prospect something tangible, a taste of your services, to close the sale. You can do this for free, or for a reduced fee. Many trainers offer a shortened training session, usually around 1/2 hour in duration, during which they provide quality training and use the time wisely to develop a good relationship with a future client.

The best way to build that relationship is by utilizing communication skills. Begin by listening to your clients, not just to what they say or how it's said (body language), but watch their mood. What were they concerned about? Reflect on your responses. Are you judging them and ready to offer rapid advice? Or are you aware that most people simply want to be listened to, nothing more? You can just let them know you heard what they said by paraphrasing (e.g., "Meg, can I tell you what I just heard so I can make sure I got it?") or by giving nonverbal cues, like nodding your head while you look at them.

This kind of deep listening and nonjudgmental response is particularly useful if clients tell you about personal matters. You can reassure them that you heard what they said and gently steer the conversation back to a professional level. It is also crucial to your success as a personal trainer, because no matter how competent you are in training, if you can't listen to your clients, it wil be much more difficult to market yourself and to build strong relationships.

Listening is also the key to building good relationships with various targets. For example, professional people typically have demanding schedules, which may include travel, and believe they don't have time to exercise or feel uncomfortable eating lowfat foods at a client dinner. To address these concerns, you may need to be flexible in your times of meeting with them and to provide them with simple yet effective ideas about how to stay active and eat well at business meals.

Suppose you want to build your business by setting up a network of referral sources, for example, nutritionists or physical therapists. Again, the best way to develop that relationship is to listen to the concerns of other professionals and offer them a win–win proposal. Put yourself in their shoes: Why would I, if I were a physical therapist, want to refer clients to a personal trainer? Am I overworked? Bored, from repetition or lack of challenge? Underpaid? Create a solution to solve their problems.

If you ever have dissatisfied clients, the best way to prevent bad word-of-mouth is to let them know you understand that they are dissatisfied. Simply listen to all their gripes without response or defending yourself for as long as they need to talk about it. The client may still choose not to work with you, but probably won't complain about you to someone else.

Develop a Creative Marketing Plan

By asking yourself the questions driven by the traditional marketing plan, including what you will offer, to whom, how, and where, you have completed about 80% of the work required to be successful in marketing yourself. This is because in asking yourself what specialty you are passionate about and what name to give your business, for example, you have already been creative. The focus of this section is to ask you to broaden your perspective and to see opportunities that others miss.

According to Paul Hawken, author of *Growing a Business*, "Good (business) ideas . . . do not look very good at first or even second glance, but don't worry if your business ideas sound weird, crazy or obscure. Like a puppy, many good ideas are awkward, helpless, and unimpressive" (Hawken, 1987). I contend that the same axiom applies to marketing.

Look at Ben & Jerry's Ice Cream. A traditional marketing plan suggested that the best markets for selling ice cream were college towns in warm climates. But when Ben and Jerry visited those locations, they found a lot of other ice cream vendors were already there. Too crowded, they decided, and headed north to Burlington, Vermont, where there wasn't a single Baskin-Robbins outlet. That was in 1978. Business was great—until winter. It looked, as Hawken said, helpless. Their only hope of survival was to package their ice cream and sell it wholesale.

As a multimillion-dollar company now with national distribution, Ben and Jerry realized they needed more than just packaging their ice cream. Consider their creativity in developing flavors, Chunky Monkey or Cherry Garcia, for example, and the way they made their first public offering of stock—by printing it on the tops of their ice cream containers.

So you say, I'm not Ben and Jerry! That's not the point. If you plan to be successful marketing your business, especially as the market you serve becomes more competitive and sophisticated, you need to be creative.

Roger von Oech has written several books, including *A Kick in the Seat of the Pants* (von Oech, 1986) and *A Whack on the Side of the Head* (von Oech, 1983), in which he argues, "If creative thinking was an important survival skill in the 1980's, it's even more important in the nineties (and beyond)." Let's just look at a few of von Oech's creativity-generating ideas.

Compare ideas: Let's say you decide to advertise your services in the classified advertising section of the local newspaper because the ad representative at the paper says it is the most cost-effective way to reach your target. Using von Oech's suggestion, compare this idea to others with that same ad person: Are there any special sections on health coming up this year that would attract a special readership who would be particularly interested in my services? Which section(s) of the paper receives the most readership on the dates I plan to advertise? Does the editorial staff know about the special type of training I provide and how I help Dr. B's patients? Would reporters appreciate receiving photos or quotes for a feature about me? Are there other potential health-related advertisers who would be interested in sharing the cost of a large ad? What else could the newspaper do to generate maximum exposure and readership for my ad (complimentary art design, special placement)?

Compare a newspaper ad to other vehicles. What other printed materials do your clients read? A health newsletter from their HMO or doctor? A billing from the electric company? The church newsletter? A brochure they picked up in a coffee shop? Something else may be less expensive and unexpected enough to generate a larger-than-usual response.

Cross-fertilize: If you need a new marketing idea, talk with people who are in totally different fields about the creative marketing approaches that have worked for them. The key here is not to reject any of their ideas outright, because even those that seem ridiculous may generate a new idea for you.

For example, consider talking with a dance instructor or a driver's education teacher. The dance instructor got new students by hanging up tap and ballet shoes for kids to try on in the local bowling alley and then gave a free class demonstration on family bowling night. This gives you a new idea: Go to the local library and bookstores and give free talks on family fitness, promoting yourself by letting the kids play with your Dynabands and medicine balls (this is a "pull" strategy, encouraging the kids to talk their parents into hiring you). The driver's education teacher complained about having to sit in a car for long, stressful periods, so you develop a creative program for in-car exercises and relaxation techniques that you can sell to other driving instructors.

These are just two strategies, comparison and cross-fertilization, to help you become more creative in your marketing efforts. If you need more help in thinking creatively, read von Oech's books, or ask a group of associates and friends who aren't in your business to help you brainstorm for unique ways to market yourself and your business. Just think, you could hold an annual business brainstorming party in January where everyone could get many new ideas for marketing their businesses.

Wherever you get your ideas, the intent of this chapter is to kickstart you toward developing the most creative and strategically smart marketing plan for your personal training business!

Summary

In this chapter, we defined basic marketing, marketing tools, and selling terms. These are necessary so just as you have a deeper understanding of "abduction" and "adduction," for example, than the average person, you'll be able to talk intelligently with other professionals and advertisers about marketing. If you take the time to utilize the worksheets and practice the selling skills, you will be smarter about how you spend your time and money to generate business and about how you describe your work. And finally, let yourself be a learner and read some of the books I've mentioned and gain further insights into yourself and your business potential. As Paul Hawken says, "the successful business is an expression of an individual person: *you*!" (Hawken, 1987).

References

Hawken, P. (1987). *Growing a business*. New York: Simon & Schuster.

Jamiel, A. (1993, Nov./Dec.). The specialist's strategy to build a client base. *IDEA Personal Trainer Newsletter*, pp. 1-3.

Rippe, J.M., & Ward, C.A. (1989). *The Rockport walking program*. New York: Prentice Hall.

Rothenberg, B., & Rothenberg, O. (1994). *Touch training for strength*. Champaign, IL: Human Kinetics.

Seligman, M.E.P. (1991). *Learned optimism*. New York: Alfred A. Knopf.

von Oech, R. (1983). *A whack on the side of the head*. New York: Warner Books.

von Oech, R. (1986). *A kick in the seat of the pants*. Toronto: Fitzhenry & Whiteside.

Chapter 6

Managing Your Personal Training Business

Gregory J. Florez

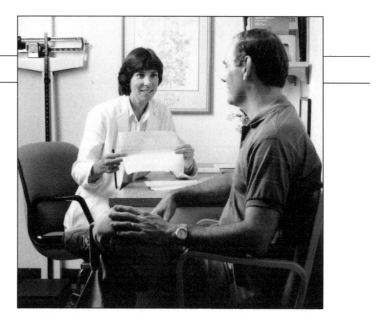

The objectives of this chapter are to

- discuss the importance of a personal vision for yourself and a mission statement for your business,
- discuss how to hire staff members and train your trainers, and
- discuss compensation for employees.

Overview

Managing a business is both an art and a science. You may have heard the phrase *good leaders are born, not made.* To some degree this is true. Obtaining an MBA does not guarantee that you will be a good leader. Leading people or running a business requires good communication skills, business skills, and a host of other talents. One thing is certain: Managing is not easy, especially if it's your own business. Owning or managing your own business requires making difficult decisions often. This chapter presents essential information on how to manage a personal training business effectively. Whether you work alone or you decide to open a personal training company and hire employees, good leadership skills are essential for success.

Before you consider how to run your personal training business, it is important to take a look at how you want to run your life. Sound strange? Consider this. You will spend a great deal of your time and energy working on your business. If you are successful, your business wil thrive, creating new opportunities and also new stresses and problems to solve. There comes a point when all successful business owners must decide what they want their company to look like and do. I believe that in order to make this decision, you must be absolutely sure of your personal vision. Keep in mind that this is your business, not your whole life. If you can look at working *on* your business, rather than *in* your business, you will create a better personal training business. Remember that your business is an entity unto itself. It has its own needs and momentum, separate from your own personal needs.

You must first define a vision of what you want your life to look like. In his book *The E Myth*, Michael Gerber helps entrepreneurs understand these distinctions in order to help themselves establish clear goals for their businesses and their lives. Do you want to build a business that you run on your own? Do you want to hire employees? Private contractors? Possibly take on a partner? How much money do you need to make? Do you have a family? How much free time is important to you? Answering questions like these will give you some help in determining a direction for yourself. The answers will form the foundation for how you manage and grow your business. I believe that if you do not enjoy the process of managing your business, you will never create a business that will grow and prosper in the long term.

Mission Statement

As noted in chapter 4, a mission statement will help you focus on your beliefs about how to run your business. It also creates a sense of purpose and credibility when you share your mission statement with your clients and prospective clients. And it will remind you of your vision and goals if you suffer a lapse in confidence. Make it a simple and truthful statement about what you want to provide for your customers: it should be concise and communicate your purpose clearly. You should be proud to share your mission with your clients and other business associates. I thought it might be helpful to share my company's first mission statement (as a company, we have made changes to our mission statement as we have grown and had more employees contribute to its meaning).

Each one of us at First Fitness is committed to providing the highest level of service to each client in the areas of fitness consultation, personal training, nutrition consultation, listening, and facilitation in the health and wellness field. We promise to provide any tools necessary to help empower our clients and help them take action to improve all aspects of their physical and mental lifestyles, whether they are corporations, health clubs, or individuals.

Our mission statement reflects that First Fitness is a sizable company for our industry, providing diverse services to a variety of clients. It may be too broad for a smaller company or single trainer operation.

Client Policies

Client policies are much more than just written forms and methods of doing business. They help define your business and create an organized structure on which clients and trainers can rely. Sound business policies are also critical to your cash flow, long-term financial stability, and credibility with your clients. Inconsistent or nonexistent client policies are very prevalent in our industry. If personal training is truly to be a growth industry with many successful companies and trainers, we must all implement good business practices.

There are many resources available that will provide you with the forms and mechanical tools to provide consistent policies. Look into products sold in periodicals or books, at personal training workshops and trade shows, and professional groups like Personal Training Resources. Chapter 4 lists sound guidelines for billing and cancellation policies and client documentation. A sample billing agreement is shown in Figure 6.1 and a sample medical clearance form appears in Figure 6.2.

Hiring Staff Members

At some point you may decide to hire additional staff members. Working one-on-one with clients is labor intensive, and if you truly care about and value your clients, it can be mentally draining as well. Adding trainers is a natural progression in the business of personal training. Hiring and training additional staff members gives you the opportunity to increase your income, and of course, grow your business. It also provides additional challenges and helps you develop new skills.

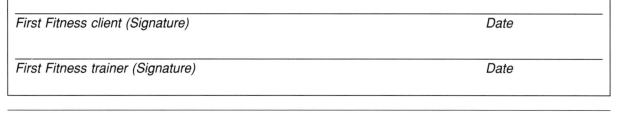

Billing Agreement

First Fitness bills its personal fitness training clients on a prepay basis. Bills are issued directly to a client by a trainer and are due upon receipt.

First Fitness trainers work on a scheduled appointment basis. In order for us to effectively use our time, we ask that clients give trainers a 24-hour notice when canceling an appointment. This means a cancellation should be made at least 24 hours before the scheduled appointment. Personal training sessions canceled inside of 24 hours of the scheduled appointment will be billed at the normal rate of a single session. All canceled appointments outside the 24-hour time frame must be made up within that scheduled week in order to receive credit for the session.

I, _____, have read the billing agreement and accept these policies as they relate to personal fitness training procedures with my First Fitness personal trainer.

_____
First Fitness client (Signature)   *Date*

_____
First Fitness trainer (Signature)   *Date*

Figure 6.1   Sample billing agreement.

Interviewing

It's been said that great businesses are built not by extraordinary people, but by ordinary people doing extraordinary work. I have found this to be true. It is sound business practice to use interviewing and hiring techniques that give you the very best chance of hiring candidates who most closely fit the needs of your business. I strongly believe that there are some traits that a candidate must possess, because some behaviors cannot be taught. But there are traits that a candidate does not necessarily need as a prerequisite because you can provide adequate training in these areas once he or she is hired. There is much conjecture as to what can be trained and what must be hired. (See Table 6.1 for some examples based on my experience in recruiting trainers.) These are two very short lists that parallel some of the skills needed in a good personal trainer. Keep in mind that in order to train new hires in a particular area (from the can-be-trained group), you must commit your resources. You must allow ample time to train your new trainers.

There are many methods for screening and hiring candidates. One that I have used with success is a format that examines a candidate's past behaviors. Its premise is that people display consistent behaviors from one work environment to the next. Early in the hiring process, the interviewer determines how the candidate has behaved in previous jobs. The questions are directed toward behaviors that you know to be important for success in your business.

Let's use an example: You run a small personal training business with trainers who train in homes and other settings, collect money, and manage their own schedules. In short, they are very autonomous. You know that your trainers must demonstrate the behavior of taking control of a situation. You might ask this question: "Jody, tell me about a situation, in work or school, where you were working with a team or group that was not meeting its deadlines or working well toward its goal. I'd like to know specifically how you handled the situation." You are looking for an answer that demonstrates how the candidate took control of the situation, made decisions that helped the group, and tried to get it back

Table 6.1   Trainer Skills

Can be trained	Must be hired
Technical skills	Initiative
Exercise testing skills	Taking ownership of clients
Hands-on training techniques	Adaptability
Sales presentation skills	Goal orientation
Listening skills	

Medical Clearance Form

Your patient, _____ , has applied to participate in one-on-one training with *First Fitness, Inc.,* which requires your medical clearance prior to participation. Clearance indicates that this patient has no contraindications for participation in the fitness tests described below and one-on-one training. The patient will have the following tests administered to determine his or her state of fitness.

1) Health risk appraisal/questionnaire
2) Resting measures (i.e., heart rate, blood pressure, % body fat, anthropometrics)
3) Muscle strength/endurance assessment
4) Cardiorespiratory assessment
5) Flexibility assessment

Some organizations recommend that an individual over 40 years of age who has not been involved in an exercise program on a regular basis have a diagnostic exercise test prior to beginning such a program. Does your patient's risk factor assessment warrant such a test prior to beginning his or her program? _____ Yes _____ No

My patient, _____ , is physically able to participate in the testing regimen described above and in a vigorous, individually instructed exercise program.

Signature: _____ M.D.

Address: _____

_____
| City | State | Zip |

Please list any restrictions or concerns (including medications). Thank you for your cooperation.

_____

_____

_____

_____

Please return medical clearance form to:

First Fitness, Inc.
2000 N. Racine Suite 3800
Chicago, IL 60614

Figure 6.2 Sample medical clearance.

---

on track. Always keep the candidate directed toward specifics and try to find out only what he or she did.

Candidates will often speak in terms of *we,* making it difficult to find out what their specific role was. Keep prodding them to explain their personal role. You'll find that you don't have to dig to find the behavior that you are looking for. It will usually jump out at you when you ask real-life, situational questions similar to the example. Identify four or five key behaviors that are most important to you and build questions around them.

One other point needs to be made regarding recruiting and hiring: Although we see ourselves as exercise specialists, our technical qualifications are only a part of what is necessary to manage and grow a successful personal training business. Many outstanding trainers are not successful on their own because they lack the business savvy and management skills to make personal training a full-time career. You need to hire good technical trainers, but you also need people who know how to sell, recruit, and manage the business side of your company.

Trainer Status

Hiring part-time versus full-time employees is a major consideration when you decide to add staff members. Each has it advantages and disadvantages. Part-time employees work less hours, consequently saving the company payroll, Social Security taxes, and associated tax consulting costs. The company also saves the expense of providing benefits like health insurance, workman's compensation, and paid vacations normally afforded its full-time employees. Essentially, a part-time worker is a part-time provider of services to your corporation. You may pay a part-time worker a salary or hourly rate. Taxes are withheld according to the amount paid per paycheck.

Part-time employees may supplement their income with another job. In many situations, this other job will be personal training with their own client base. Make sure your employment contracts for part-time employees specify restrictions against acquiring any of your company's clients or referrals if the employee is discharged or leaves.

Hiring full-time employees represents a very different accounting relationship. You are responsible for keeping and filing proper taxation forms (W-4, etc.). Your company must also deduct correct withholding amounts from employee paychecks, provide quarterly tax reports to the IRS, and keep detailed payroll records. You must also provide workman's compensation. As an employer, you are responsible for a portion of your employees' Social Security taxes as well as unemployment compensation taxes, expenses that will affect your bottom line. You are more restrained by law when terminating the employment of an employee. You have authority to supervise, direct work volume, and evaluate trainers who are your employees. Hiring employees also can create a better foundation for a long-term relationship.

Professional liability insurance must be provided for all part-time and full-time employees. IDEA provides this type of insurance at $1 million per employee with very competitive group rates. It works out to be about $60 to $90 per full-time employee per year. If you have part-time employees, every two are counted as one full-time employee. In addition, you will receive a discount if any of your people are ACE certified or have a 4-year degree in an exercise field. The monetary amount you agree to cover each employee is up to you. Since your company will be paying part or all of the bill, the remainder can be taken out of the employee's paycheck via payroll deductions.

A successful way to begin a relationship may be to start a trainer as a part-time employee, with the ability to move into a full-time employment opportunity. This gives you some freedom as an employer to be able to evaluate a trainer as a part-time employee before making a commitment. It is important that

you structure and give very clear guidelines to new part-time employees, showing them the path to become full-time workers. I've outlined a sample scenario below:

1. Part-time trainer is hired and paid a percentage of all personally billed training hours.
2. Guidelines for number of clients retained, referrals, and so on are established in order for the part-time trainer to reach the next level.
3. Performance is reviewed at 60 days using specific guidelines outlined in initial job offer. At this time a percentage increase in pay might be warranted.
4. When a predetermined number of weekly training hours is reached, the trainer has the opportunity to become a full-time salaried employee with benefits (e.g., trainer is paid an annual salary of $25,000 for training 20 hours per week). It is important that the trainer actually maintain a training schedule of 20 hours per week before becoming a full-time, salaried employee.
5. Trainer's performance is reviewed periodically. If weekly average drops below 20 hours for a significant period of time, the salary and employment status are subject to review and renegotiation.

Giving new trainers the opportunity to become full-time employees and the ability to advance in the company is critical. If you are interested in growing your business, it is important to show good trainers a path to success. You must be able to help the trainer move to full-time status. Again, it is important to have advice from an attorney and accountant in setting up guidelines for hiring and creating a basic payroll system for your growing business.

Commissions and Bonuses

Whether you employ a staff of trainers or hire part-time employees, it is important to motivate them to help you continue to grow your business and provide a good income for themselves. New clients will use your services because of referrals from others and solicitations from your own trainers. Having your trainers actively ask for referral leads from their current clients and other contacts is a low-cost, effective way to increase your client base. It is important to have your trainers share in the responsibility and success of bringing new clients and generating revenue for your business. Providing commissions to your trainers will help increase business and provide trainers with specific ways to increase their income.

The amount of commission and any bonus structure that you set up are completely dependent on your company's financial situation, costs of doing business, margins, and pay arrangements with your trainers.

Pay Structures

Assuming that you are either hiring your trainers as part-time or full-time employees, let's look at a few sample pay structures. I would strongly recommend asking an accountant for guidance.

Pay for part-time employees should be kept very simple. You pay a trainer a specific fee or a percentage of a client fee for providing a specific service. The amount that you pay to a part-time trainer for a personal training session will vary depending on individual competence, education, and experience. It is my strong belief that, in addition to compensation for services performed, part-time trainers should earn commissions when they bring new clients or sell other services and products for your company.

Hiring employees creates a more structured format for increasing your staff. Explore the possibility of providing full-time salaried employment to trainers who excel because this will help your business grow. If you are serious about growing a company and creating a supportive, committed staff, this is a step that is absolutely necessary at some point. You must show a logical progression toward full-time employment. Trainers start as part-time employees, paid for only the work that they generate and bill. Let's say that you pay trainers at the rate of 50% for all of their personal training sessions. The next step is to give them a goal to bill a certain number of hours each week. When they can maintain the desired work load with the client base, you advance them to full-time salary status.

Two things are very important in this progression. The weekly number of hours for salary status must be realistic (for both the company and the trainer), and trainers must understand their responsibility to meet that goal—very specifically. Here's a plan for advancement:

Part-time trainer

- Trainer earns 50% of the total fee for a training hour up to 20 hours per week. Trainer consistently works at 20 hours per week for a 2-month period.

Trainer becomes full time

- Trainer advances to full-time annual salary of $25,000 for a 20-hour training week.

- Trainer receives a bonus of 60% of the total fee for a training hour for all hours over 20 trained per week.

- Trainer is reviewed on a quarterly basis. If average training week drops below 20 hours, the trainer is subject to a salary renegotiation (possibly reverting back to part-time level).

This is one scenario that works well, with one particular caveat. It must be managed constantly. You need to have a system in place to monitor your trainers' weekly schedules. This means not only their current hours, but also their projected hours. In our business, many clients who can afford this service are also able to leave for lengthy periods of time during holidays, summers, and so on. This creates gaps (often seasonal) in the availability of hours for your trainers. Salaried-trainer schedules must be managed ahead of time to plan for these fluctuations. With this projected information, trainers can work toward prospecting for new clients, committing other clients to more days per week, and use other methods for filling in those lost hours. In this respect, having a multitrainer organization is advantageous because trainers can help each other out with clients during seasonal lows.

You should also plan to provide additional incentives and benefits to full-time salaried employees as you grow. Although there is a cost to benefits, costs can be offset by using benefits as part of an overall compensation package. Some possible benefits might include

- car phone reimbursement for trainers who sell and travel,
- health care insurance,
- professional liability insurance,
- workman's compensation insurance
- bonuses for exceeding training goals,
- continued education benefits, and
- certification and workshop reimbursement.

Training the Trainer

In a business where you are asked to provide a skilled personal service to a variety of clients, *training the trainer* is a key to continued success. As a trainer you probably have some valuable skills in areas that relate to working one-on-one with clients in providing exercise testing and prescription (a prescribed, logical progression of exercise and goal setting for your clients). Depending on your background, you may or may not be skilled in other areas that are important to successful management of a personal training business. These include

- business development skills/referrals,
- client retention,
- listening and facilitation skills, and
- dealing with client conflict, adherence, and failure.

These are all important skills for every trainer to learn and use on a continuing basis. Conferences and workshops can give you a good foundation for dealing with diverse issues. You should also offer a program for ongoing internal training so that everyone involved with your organization can improve their skills. Training is valuable, and there are a variety of methods to help you train your staff. Some training techniques that we have used and found to be extremely effective include role playing, videotaping, written exercises, client feedback, and workshops.

Role Playing

Using dyads, triads, and small-group workshops, a business owner will set up and facilitate role-playing workshops based on simulated trainer–client interactions. This type of training is very effective in helping trainers handle real-life situations that occur when they are one-on-one with clients. Simply put, a business owner needs to construct situations that parallel those happening in the business environment, including

- new client consultations,
- cancellation–conflict situations,
- dissatisfied/irate clients,
- sales calls,
- client follow-up phone calls, and
- asking for client referrals.

Let me give you an example of how to set up a role play to train a trainer to ask for client referrals. You will need two people for this exercise, the trainer and someone to play the part of the client. Prior to the training, give the trainer an outline or script highlighting the key points in asking for a referral. Depending on the background and skill level of your trainer, the script may use exact phrases or it may cover key points only. Here is a sample script (using only key points) for asking clients for referrals.

- Ask clients to spend a few minutes with you after a training session.
- Thank them for their continued support of you and your business.

- Let them know that you have some additional openings in your schedule.
- Ask them if they know anyone who can benefit from your services.
- Ask for a name and phone number and permission to call the referral.
- Thank them for the referral (a note or card is a good idea).
- If you give clients a free session, t-shirt, or other item in return for a referral, complete the act.
- Contact the referral.

This is a skeleton script for referral sales. Depending upon the skill level of those being trained, you can customize it and add detail to each point. Using the script, work with each trainer and role-play through the script, with each of you assuming your respective roles. Reverse roles—putting the trainer in both the client and trainer roles is a powerful tool when used correctly. Here is an example of how this might flow:

Trainer: *Mrs. Ross, do you have a few minutes after our session today? There is something I'd like to ask you.*

Client: *Yes, I have an extra 5 minutes.*

(At end of session) **Trainer:** *We have been working together for 5 months now and have discussed your progress, and also your future goals. I appreciate the fact that you have told me you feel it is going so well and are enjoying the training. I've enjoyed working with you and appreciate your support and interest. I have some additional openings in my schedule and wonder if you know anyone who can benefit from my training.*

Client: *Actually, yes. I have a friend who has been asking about personal training. I get so focused when we're training that I forget until after you've left. I'm not sure if she wants to spend the money or knows exactly how it works.*

Trainer: *I understand. Many people don't really know how our services work. I will be happy to call her and set up a complimentary consultation. Would you mind giving her name and phone number?*

Client: *No, that would be fine. Let me give it to you.*

Trainer: *May I use your name when I call?*

Client: *Yes, of course.*

Trainer: *I really appreciate your trust in my services. As you know, this business has been built entirely by clients like you who refer their friends and family. I'll make sure that I personally follow through with your friend.*

Make sure that you personally and appropriately acknowledge your client for the referral. Sending a thank-you card or providing them with a complimentary session are good ideas. The above role play is an example that went perfectly. You will want to create scenarios that are more challenging, and always review the role-play scenario with the trainer. Use your personal experience to devise the situations. Discuss each point, give guidance and affirmation, and let the trainer begin to figure out better ways of acting through the next one. Role playing can be a powerful teaching tool, especially with employees who have limited experience in client contact.

Videotaping

Videotaping your training sessions, including role plays and lectures, will give you excellent feedback on how you and your staff are perceived in any situation, whether it be a client personal training session or a new-client consultation. As with the role-playing sessions, you want to spend additional time reviewing each taped session and debriefing the trainer. Use each session as a positive teaching tool, providing both positive feedback and also pointing out areas that need improvement. If you don't own a video camera, you can probably borrow one from a friend or rent one from a college audio-visual department or large camera store. It is worth your time to try this method. Visual and auditory feedback add a new dimension to training, as many of us never get a chance to see how we perform in a one-on-one situation.

Written Exercises

A variety of written tools allow you to sharpen the communication skills of you and your trainers. Some of these help determine how you currently deal with business and personal situations and give you specific guidance for changing your methods, based on the written evaluations. Check the business section of a large bookstore for workbooks. Other sources include large training organizations such as Skill Path and Covey Leadership Center.

Client Feedback

Using client feedback as a tool to help improve your skills and enhance your services is extremely useful. Regardless of the methods you use to gather information, all client feedback should be summarized and used to train for improved performance.

Examples of client feedback tools include the following:

- Written surveys mailed directly to the client. Surveys can be anonymous and should ask specific questions regarding their satisfaction with your services.
- Phone surveys. Call clients on a regular basis to determine their satisfaction with your services. To make your survey results more useful and standardized, use a script and ask consistent questions.
- Focus groups. Taking a sampling of clients from your company to lunch on a quarterly basis can be an excellent opportunity to really listen and get feedback on an informal basis.

Workshops

Our industry increasingly offers excellent targeted workshops and conferences to provide personal trainers with advanced information, techniques, and training advice to help them in their personal training businesses. Many organizations also provide audiotapes, videotapes, training manuals, and other materials to supplement the information given in the conference. Encourage all your trainers to review these materials on a regular basis. To make this type of training effective you must have a system of accountability in place. For instance, you might make a "Working With Postinjury Clients" videotape required viewing for your staff trainers. Develop a checkout system with a time frame for them to review the tape. Hold a general meeting to discuss the tape and determine their understanding of the material. Depending on the size of your business and the relevance of the information, you might even administer a written quiz to your trainers.

Another suggestion is to ask trainers to attend a workshop or review a tape and then conduct an in-house training session on what they learned. Another very cost-effective method of getting the most out of a workshop format is to send a trainer to a national or regional conference that has information of interest to you. Part of your agreement is that the trainer will learn the information from the conference and design a summary workshop to present to the rest of your staff. Give the trainer very specific guidelines as to your expectations, including time formats, and outline parameters, so that you ensure the presentation to your group is successful. This method not only makes financial sense, but is also rewarding for your trainers because they learn to speak in front of groups, learn how to train groups more effectively, and help grow the company. Be creative, but realize that you must develop ways to determine whether these types of training methods are effective.

A valuable lesson to learn is that initial training of any kind is just that—initial training. You need to work on your skills (and the skills of everyone on your staff) constantly. If you are committed to providing training for yourself and your staff, reviewing and improving formats continually, you will see steady progress in the areas in which you train.

Managing for the Long Haul

It's been said that for businesses to survive they must grow steadily and constantly. Although I initially disagreed with that philosophy, I now believe it to be true. To keep good people you must establish goals (i.e., show them a path) and then provide the means to achieve them. You must also decide what you want your life to look like and keep that picture in mind as your business grows. If you don't stay fresh and excited, your business will surely reflect that.

The fitness training business is very labor intensive, and you will need to work with others who share your vision and commitment to fuel your growth. You need others to help you build and create a shared vision. These people need to be compensated competitively and given continued opportunities to accept new challenges and grow. More importantly, they need to be acknowledged and made to feel important. This process is a personal one and must be done in an honest, meaningful way. That is the essence of a company, especially in a

personal business where we provide specialized services. You cannot do the job alone!

Personal training businesses are very logical, but not simple. Successful companies will learn the essentials:

1. Finding and keeping clients
2. Finding and keeping good trainers
3. Helping clients get continuous benefit
4. Continually training and empowering staff members

Keeping these essentials in mind (and adding your own personal goals) and structuring your business around them will help create the foundation for your success.

Summary

This chapter is about managing a personal training company. Expertise and certification are absolutely essential. The consumer is becoming more knowledgeable and sophisticated, even as the industry becomes flooded with new trainers. Decide what you do best, and do it—better than anyone else. Continue to educate yourself and your trainers. Successful trainers need to develop some basic client recruitment tools and skills and learn to listen to their clients.

Hiring and managing good people is a full-time job. Continually training them is essential, not only to the success of the company, but also to nurture your employees and create leaders for the future. If you are like most personal training business owners, you started by yourself, training one client at a time. At some point you need to identify competent individuals, teach them how you work, and give them specific responsibilities. Let them come up with ideas on their own, take risks, and earn rewards. Finally, be ready to step back and let them help you run your company.

Chapter 7

Legal and Professional Responsibilities of Personal Training

David L. Herbert

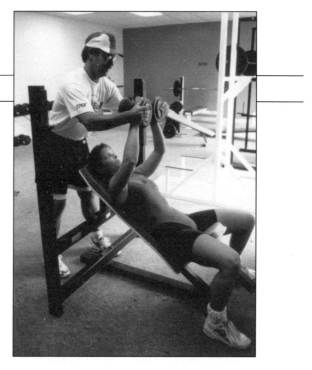

The objectives of this chapter are to

- discuss the standard of care for personal trainers,
- review basic legal terms as they apply to personal trainers, and
- define the unauthorized practice of medicine and allied health care.

Overview

Understanding the legal aspects of personal training cannot be overlooked. We live in a very litigious society, and certainly personal trainers are not excluded in any way from legal problems. Every personal trainer needs to understand the legal aspects involved in the creation and operation of a personal training business. The more you understand about the laws that pertain to your trade, the better you'll be able to reduce the risk of legal problems. This chapter presents a review of the important legal aspects of personal training. All aspects of your personal training business should be evaluated from a legal standpoint. Personal trainers should never take the legal aspects of their trade lightly.

The delivery of personal training services to consumers by a variety of professionals has grown rapidly in the last decade. The demand for such services has been so great that many professionals, including physical therapists, chiropractors, athletic trainers, strength and conditioning coaches, and exercise specialists have entered this domain. Those primarily delivering services to individual clients in one-on-one or small-group settings include licensed and nonlicensed, as well as association-certified and noncertified, personal trainers.

No hard and fast legal rules have been developed for the personal training service explosion. Many within this industry simply plunged into business without a thorough appreciation of their legal and professional responsibilities. Active personal trainers and those about to enter the business have to know and understand certain general legal and professional responsibilities associated with personal training activities (Koeberle, 1990).

The Standard of Care for Personal Trainers

Personal trainers, like all other service providers, are required by law to deliver service in accordance with the so-called standard of care. Deviations from the expected standard of care are often subject to personal injury actions based upon claims of negligence against trainers by clients who are injured due to alleged substandard care. Negligence may be defined as failure to conform one's conduct to a generally accepted standard or duty, which proximately causes harm to an individual to whom the former owed some duty or responsibility. While lay jurors often judge deficiencies in regard to care delivery, "expert witnesses" may testify to the expected standard of care. In contested cases, expert witnesses are allowed to offer testimony as to claimed deviations from that standard of care (or adherence to it) based upon their educational backgrounds, training, and experience. The purpose of such testimony is to educate jurors as to provider norms for the delivery of care.

In years past, expert witnesses often offered opinions based on their own individual training and experience. Many times conflicting statements by a number of experts led to inconsistent verdicts. Consequently, it was often difficult for trainers to protect themselves from attack and criticism in a court of law.

Today, many professional practice domains, including personal training, have developed written standards of practice to assist in defining the breadth and scope of their practices. Personal trainers must ensure that they deliver service in accordance with the expected professional standard of care. It is important for trainers to realize that professionally derived and expressed *standards of care*, *guidelines*, *recommendations*, or *parameters of practice* are the expected norm for professional behavior and are likely to be used in conjunction with litigation to assess and compare trainers' conduct. Such a process will be used in the event of litigation to judge or evaluate questions related to whether or not care or service was properly provided to an individual client by the defendant trainer. In order to fully appreciate this process, trainers need to be thoroughly familiar with the expressed standard-of-care statements that have been developed by, among others, the National Strength and Conditioning Association (NSCA), the American Council on Exercise (ACE), and the American College of Sports Medicine (ACSM). Guidelines for exercise testing, lists of coronary risk factors, and any other set of safety standards are considered to be standard-of-care statements. For example, Figure 7.1 shows the ACSM's standards for contraindications to exercise testing. Trainers can use these expressed standards statements to prospectively define how they will deliver service to clients. Adherence to industry standards will also minimize the importance of expert testimony should claim and litigation ever arise.

Certified or advanced trainers (especially those who hold higher competency certifications) should know and appreciate that according to most standards statements, they will probably be held to a standard of care greater than that required for other fitness providers. As a consequence, holders of higher credentials or certifications will be expected to deliver care according to those higher standards.

Personal Trainers' Duties and Responsibilities

Personal trainers have a number of duties and responsibilities inherent in the delivery of service to clients. Deviations in any of these areas may well be actionable and lead to injury claims and lawsuits.

Health Screening

Among the most important of their duties, personal trainers have an obligation to screen clients for activity, to recommend and lead activity, and to supervise exercise in accord with established guidelines.

Absolute Contraindications

1. A recent significant change in the resting ECG suggesting infarction or other acute cardiac events
2. Recent complicated myocardial infarction
3. Unstable angina
4. Uncontrolled ventricular dysrhythmia
5. Uncontrolled atrial dysrhythmia that compromises cardiac function
6. Third-degree A-V block
7. Acute congestive heart failure
8. Severe aortic stenosis
9. Suspected or known dissecting aneurysm
10. Active or suspected myocarditis or pericarditis
11. Thrombophlebitis or intracardiac thrombi
12. Recent systemic or pulmonary embolus
13. Acute infection
14. Significant emotional distress (psychosis)

Relative Contraindications

1. Resting diastolic blood pressure > 120 mm Hg or resting systolic blood pressure > 200 mm Hg
2. Moderate valvular heart disease
3. Known electrolyte abnormalities (hypokalemia, hypomagnesemia)
4. Fixed-rate pacemaker (rarely used)
5. Frequent or complex ventricular ectopy
6. Ventricular aneurysm
7. Cardiomyopathy, including hypertrophic cardiomyopathy
8. Uncontrolled metabolic disease (e.g., diabetes, thyrotoxicosis, or myxedema)
9. Chronic infectious disease (e.g., mononucleosis, hepatitis, AIDS)
10. Neuromuscular, musculoskeletal, or rheumatoid disorders that are exacerbated by exercise
11. Advanced or complicated pregnancy

Figure 7.1 Example of professional standards of care.
Reprinted from American College of Sports Medicine (1991).

Screening based upon the recommendations of a number of organizations, including the American College of Sports Medicine (1991, 1992), can be used to determine if clients can participate safely in the proposed activity sessions. Another useful screening tool is the PAR-Q form (see Figure 7.2); it, or something similar, should be part of every trainer's preactivity screening process.

After conducting a thorough health screening, trainers can allow clients to participate in training sessions or defer admission pending medical approval. Failure to screen (Herbert, 1987, 1988a, 1992) or failure to require medical clearance or treatment (Herbert, 1993) can well be subject to legal action.

Informed Consent

Clients have a right to know what activities they will engage in and to be informed of the risks associated with those activities. In medicine this process is termed *informed consent*. Personal training requires similar consent; it plays an important part in the screening process. A trainer is obligated to disclose the risks associated with training activity. A client who knowingly assumes the risks of training will be legally presumed to have assumed those risks (see Figure 7.3). If a claim or suit should later arise from a training injury, proof of the client's consent can help establish the client's knowing assumption of the risks associated with activity (Herbert, 1993).

Physical Activity Readiness
Questionnaire - PAR-Q
(revised 1994)

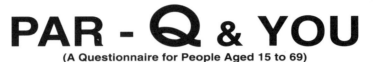

PAR - Q & YOU

(A Questionnaire for People Aged 15 to 69)

Regular physical activity is fun and healthy, and increasingly more people are starting to become more active every day. Being more active is very safe for most people. However, some people should check with their doctor before they start becoming much more physically active.

If you are planning to become much more physically active than you are now, start by answering the seven questions in the box below. If you are between the ages of 15 and 69, the PAR-Q will tell you if you should check with your doctor before you start. If you are over 69 years of age, and you are not used to being very active, check with your doctor.

Common sense is your best guide when you answer these questions. Please read the questions carefully and answer each one honestly: check YES or NO.

YES	NO		
☐	☐	1.	Has your doctor ever said that you have a heart condition <u>and</u> that you should only do physical activity recommended by a doctor?
☐	☐	2.	Do you feel pain in your chest when you do physical activity?
☐	☐	3.	In the past month, have you had chest pain when you were not doing physical activity?
☐	☐	4.	Do you lose your balance because of dizziness or do you ever lose consciousness?
☐	☐	5.	Do you have a bone or joint problem that could be made worse by a change in your physical activity?
☐	☐	6.	Is your doctor currently prescribing drugs (for example, water pills) for your blood pressure or heart condition?
☐	☐	7.	Do you know of <u>any other reason</u> why you should not do physical activity?

If

you

answered

YES to one or more questions

Talk with your doctor by phone or in person BEFORE you start becoming much more physically active or BEFORE you have a fitness appraisal. Tell your doctor about the PAR-Q and which questions you answered YES.

- You may be able to do any activity you want — as long as you start slowly and build up gradually. Or, you may need to restrict your activities to those which are safe for you. Talk with your doctor about the kinds of activities you wish to participate in and follow his/her advice.
- Find out which community programs are safe and helpful for you.

NO to all questions

If you answered NO honestly to <u>all</u> PAR-Q questions, you can be reasonably sure that you can:

- start becoming much more physically active — begin slowly and build up gradually. This is the safest and easiest way to go.
- take part in a fitness appraisal — this is an excellent way to determine your basic fitness so that you can plan the best way for you to live actively.

DELAY BECOMING MUCH MORE ACTIVE:

- if you are not feeling well because of a temporary illness such as a cold or a fever — wait until you feel better; or
- if you are or may be pregnant — talk to your doctor before you start becoming more active.

Please note: If your health changes so that you then answer YES to any of the above questions, tell your fitness or health professional. Ask whether you should change your physical activity plan.

<u>Informed Use of the PAR-Q</u>: The Canadian Society for Exercise Physiology, Health Canada, and their agents assume no liability for persons who undertake physical activity, and if in doubt after completing this questionnaire, consult your doctor prior to physical activity.

Figure 7.2   The PAR-Q.

From Canadian Society for Exercise Physiology (1994).

Personal FitnessTrainers' Sample
Express Assumption of Risk for My Participation in a Personal Fitness Training Program

I, the undersigned, hereby expressly and affirmatively state that I wish to participate in the personal fitness training program of _____ . I realize that my participation in this activity involves risk of injury, including but not limited to bodily injuries, heart attack, stroke, and even death. I also recognize that there are many other risks of injury, including serious disabling injuries, which may arise due to my participation in this activity, and that it is not possible to specifically list each and every individual injury risk. However, knowing, understanding, and appreciating the material risks and reasonably anticipating that other injuries and even death are a possibility, I hereby expressly assume all delineated risks of injury, all other possible risks of injury, and even death, which could occur by reason of my participation in this personal fitness training program.

I have also had an opportunity to ask questions. Any questions that I have asked have been answered to my complete satisfaction.

Date: _____, 19 ____.

_____
Participant

By: _____
Authorized representative

Notes of Questions and Answers

_____
_____
_____
_____

This is as stated a true and accurate record of what was asked and answered.

_____
Participant

To be checked by program staff

	Checked	Initialed
I. Risks were orally discussed.	_____	_____
II. Questions were asked, and the participant indicated complete understanding of the risks.	_____	_____
III. Questions were not asked, but an opportunity for questions was provided and the participant indicated complete understanding of the risks.	_____	_____

Date: _____, 19____ _____
Staff member

Figure 7.3 Sample assumption-of-risk form.
Reprinted from Koeberle (1990).

As part of the preactivity screening process, personal trainers may also wish to have clients sign a prospective waiver of liability or so-called release (see Figure 7.4). In some jurisdictions, properly drafted waivers of liability can be enforceable and serve to protect the personal trainer from later claim and suit.

Appropriate Activity Prescription

Personal trainers also have a clear professional duty to properly recommend or prescribe appropriate client activity, based on individual health screening and fitness assessments. Recommendations for activity must be based on professional standards and activity must be carried out within parameters set by applicable standards of practice (ACSM, 1991, 1992). Deficiencies in this process can lead to substantial claims and suits (*DeRouren v. Holiday Spa Health Clubs of California*, 1988).

Appropriate client supervision, according to accepted professional guidelines, is a required part of the standard of care for personal trainers (Koeberle, 1990). Although unsupervised activity does have a place in some programs, for some activities (Herbert & Herbert, 1993), the personal trainer service model is directed at "personal" service provision to the client in one-on-one or small-group settings necessarily involving close supervision. Consequently, personal trainers will undoubtedly be held to a legal and professional requirement to closely supervise client activity (Koeberle, 1990).

Personal trainers have an obligation to properly lead and supervise all client activity. Adherence to the previously mentioned professional standards of practice is required and constitutes the essential standard of care expected of the personal trainer.

Inspection of Facilities and Equipment

Personal trainers also have a duty to inspect areas where activity is to take place and either to make those areas safe for activity or to warn the client of areas that are not safe. It is important for trainers to recognize that service delivery takes place in a variety of settings. These settings include club-type facilities; gymnasiums; trainer-provided facilities, including mobile units; and client homes and offices. Due to the fact that services are delivered at a variety of sites, personal trainers may need to conduct several different site inspections each day to ensure that they are working in environments that are safe and free from defects or unreasonably dangerous conditions. The safety of each training site, even if it is in a client's home or office, must be judged by the trainer rather than by the client. The trainer is responsible for repairing any unsafe condition or at least warning the client as to dangerous conditions that the inspection disclosed or should have disclosed (see Figure 7.5).

Personal trainers also have a duty to inspect, maintain, and repair their equipment. Deficiencies in this regard are actionable. Failures to repair or warn users of dangerous or unrepaired equipment may also amount to willful and wanton negligence for which (in the event of client injury) the personal trainer may be subject to judicatory assessments for compensatory and punitive damages (Herbert, 1988b). Trainers must perform regular, ongoing, daily equipment inspection and weekly equipment maintenance. Adequate documentation of these efforts is also important and must be performed and maintained on a regular basis (see Figure 7.6).

Unauthorized Practice of Health Care

In all states, particular statutes exist that authorize certain licensed health care providers to render health care services. These standards govern the practice of medicine, nursing, chiropractic, physical therapy, and (in some jurisdictions) athletic training. The unauthorized practice of health care by those who are not appropriately licensed is proscribed and can result in criminal prosecution or a finding of elevated responsibility where a client is injured and suit results (*Stetina v. State Medical Licensing Board*, 1987).

Personal trainers must not cross into areas reserved for licensed practitioners. As a general rule, so long as activity, exercise, or counseling is not used to "treat," "cure," or "prevent" a disease process, condition, or injury, no violation of these laws would probably occur (Herbert & Herbert, 1993). Personal trainers should consult their lawyers to determine the existence and extent of such laws in their states.

Agreement and Release of Liability

1. In consideration of being allowed to participate in the personal fitness training activities and programs of _____ and to the use of its facilities, equipment, and services, in addition to the payment of any fee or charge, I do hereby forever waive, release, and discharge _____ and its officers, agents, employees, representatives, executors, and all others acting on their behalf from any and all claims or liabilities for injuries or damages to my person and/or property, including those caused by the negligent act or omission of any of those mentioned or others acting on their behalf, arising out of or connected with my participation in any activities, programs, or services of _____, or the use of any equipment at various sites, including home, provided by and/or recommended by _____. (*Please initial ____*)

2. I have been informed, understand, and am aware that strength, flexibility, and aerobic exercises, including the use of equipment, are potentially hazardous activities. I also have been informed, understand, and am aware that fitness activities involve a risk of injury, including a remote risk of death or serious disability, and that I am voluntarily participating in these activities and using equipment and machinery with full knowledge, understanding, and appreciation of the dangers involved. I hereby agree to expressly assume and accept any and all risks of injury or death. (*Please initial ____*)

3. I do hereby further declare myself to be physically sound and suffering from no condition, impairment, disease, infirmity, or other illness that would prevent my participation or use of equipment or machinery. I do hereby acknowledge that I have been informed of the need for a physician's approval for my participation in the exercise activities, programs, and use of exercise equipment. I also acknowledge that it has been recommended that I have yearly or more frequent physical examinations and consultations with my physician as to physical activity, exercise, and use of exercise equipment. I acknowledge that I have either had a physical examination and have been given my physician's permission to participate, or that I have decided to participate in the exercise activities, programs, and use of equipment without the approval of my physician and do hereby assume all responsibility for my participation in said activities, programs, and use of equipment. (*Please initial ____*)

4. I understand that _____'s provision and maintenance of an exercise/fitness program for me does not constitute an acknowledgment, representation, or indication of my physiological well-being, or a medical opinion relating thereto. (*Please initial ____*)

Agreed to this _____ day of _____, 19____.

_____
Client's signature

By: _____
Authorized representative

Figure 7.4   Sample release-of-liability form.
Reprinted from Koeberle (1990).

Safety Checklist

I. Facility

A. Flooring

___ Wooden flooring on platform free of splinters, holes, protruding nails, and screws

___ Tile flooring resistant to slipping; no moisture or chalk accumulation

___ Rubber flooring free of cuts, slits, and large gaps between pieces

___ Interlocking mats secure and arranged so as not to pull apart or become deformed (no protruding tabs)

___ Carpet free of tears; wear areas protected by throw mats

___ Area swept and vacuumed or mopped on a regular basis

___ Flooring glued and fastened down properly

___ Fixed equipment attached securely to floor

B. Walls (including mirrors and windows, exits, storage areas, and shelves)

___ Walls in high-activity areas free of protruding apparatus

___ Mirrors and shelves securely fixed to walls

___ Mirrors and windows cleaned regularly (twice weekly)

___ Mirrors (if present in platform areas) minimum of 50 cm off the floor

___ Mirrors not cracked or distorted

C. Environmental factors (noise control, temperature, ventilation, humidity, lighting, electrical cords and outlets, and posted signs)

___ Volume of stereo system set low enough to allow clear communication between the spotter and lifter at all times

___ Stereo system controlled by the facility coordinator and qualified supervisors

___ Air temperature kept constant at 22° to 26° C

___ Ventilation systems working properly (minimum of 8-10 air exchanges/hr and optimally 12-15 air exchanges/hr); no detectable strong odors in the room

___ Equipment not slick due to high humidity

___ Facility well lighted and free of dark areas; bulbs changed on regular basis

___ Exit sign is well lighted

___ Extension cords are routed, secured, and grounded and large enough for electrical load

___ All safety, regulation, and policy signs posted in clear view (two or three central places within facility; more postings in large facilities)

II. Equipment

A. Aerobic/anaerobic fitness area (rowing machines, bikes, sprint machines, stair machines, skiing and climbing machines)

___ Easy access to each work station (minimum of 2 ft [61 cm] between machines: 3 ft [91 cm] optimal)

___ Bolts and screws tight

___ Functioning parts easily adjustable

___ Parts and surfaces properly lubricated and cleaned

(continued)

Figure 7.5   Sample equipment- and facility-inspection form.
From National Strength and Conditioning Association (1994).

___ Foot and body straps secure and nonripping

___ Measurement devices for tension, time, rpms, etc., properly functioning

___ Surfaces that contact human skin cleaned and disinfected daily

B. Machines area (isokinetic, variable resistance, single-station, multistation machines)

   ___ Easy access to each work station (minimum of 2 ft [61 cm] between machines; 3 ft [91 cm] optimal)

   ___ Area free of loose bolts, screws, cables, and chains

   ___ Proper pins used

   ___ Securing straps functional

   ___ Parts and surfaces properly lubricated and cleaned (guide rods on selectorized machines cleared and lubricated two or three times/week)

   ___ Protective padding free of cracks and tears

   ___ Surfaces that contact human skin cleaned and disinfected daily

   ___ All parts smoothly functioning and lubricated regularly

   ___ No protruding screws or parts that need tightening or removal

   ___ Belts, chains, and cables aligned with machine parts

   ___ No worn parts (frayed cable, loose chains, worn bolts, cracked joint screws, etc.)

C. Rehabilitation and special-population machine area

   ___ Easy access to each work station (minimum of 2 ft [61 cm] between machines; 3 ft [91 cm] optimal)

   ___ Parts and surfaces properly lubricated and cleaned

   ___ Area free of loose bolts, screws, cables, and chains

   ___ Proper use of attachments, pins, and other apparatus

   ___ Surfaces that contact human skin cleaned and disinfected daily

   ___ Securing straps functional

   ___ Protective padding free of cracks and tears

   ___ All parts smoothly functioning

   ___ No protruding screws or parts that need tightening or removal

   ___ No worn parts

D. Body-weight–resistance apparatus area (sit-up board, dips, pulleys, hyperextension benches, plyometrics boxes, medicine balls, climbing ropes, pegboard climb, jump ropes)

   ___ Apparatus properly lubricated

   ___ Surfaces that contact human skin cleaned and disinfected daily

   ___ Protective padding free of cracks and tears

   ___ Securing straps and apparatus functional

   ___ Climbing apparatus secured with well-padded floor area

   ___ Properly padded floor area below plyometrics boxes

   ___ Nonslip material on the top surface and bottom or base of plyometrics boxes

   ___ Apparatus for holding feet for sit-ups, hyperextension, etc., secure

E. Stretching area (mats, stretching sticks, medicine balls, elastic cords, wall ladders)

   ___ Mat area free of weight benches and equipment

   ___ Mats free of tears

(continued)

Figure 7.5 *(continued)*

___ No large gaps between stretching mats
___ Area swept and disinfected daily
___ Stretching sticks and medicine balls properly stored after use
___ Elastic cords secured to base with safety knot and checked for wear

F. Free-weight area (bench presses, incline presses, squat racks, dumbbells, weight racks)

___ Proper spacing of racks and weight standards to allow access to all areas
___ All equipment returned after use to avoid obstruction of pathway
___ Safety equipment (belts, collars, safety bars) used and returned
___ Protective padding free of cracks and tears
___ Surfaces that contact human skin cleaned and disinfected daily
___ Securing bolts and apparatus parts (collars, curl bars) tightly fastened
___ Nonslip mats on squat rack floor area
___ Olympic bars turn properly and are properly lubricated and tightened
___ Benches, weight racks, standards, etc., secured to the floor or wall
___ Nonfunctional or broken equipment removed from area or locked out of service

G. Lifting platform area (Olympic bars, standards, bumper plates, racks, locks, chalk bins)

___ Olympic bars properly spaced (3 feet [91 cm] between ends; lifting area is 12 × 8 ft [3.7 × 2.4 m])
___ All equipment returned after use to avoid obstruction of lifting area
___ Base on all lifting standards secured
___ Olympic bar rotates properly and is properly lubricated and tightened
___ Bent Olympic bars replaced; knurling clear of debris
___ Collars functioning
___ Sufficient chalk available to lifters
___ Wrist straps, belts, and knee wraps available, functioning, and stored properly
___ Benches, chairs, boxes kept at a distance from lifting area
___ No gaps, cuts, slits, splinters in mat
___ Area properly swept and mopped to remove splinters, chalk, etc.
___ Ceiling space sufficient for overhead lifts (12 ft [3.7 m] minimum) and free of low-hanging apparatus (beams, pipes, lighting, signs, etc.)

Figure 7.5 *(continued)*

Summary

Personal trainers have a variety of legal and professional concerns to consider within their profession. It is important for trainers to adhere to national practice statements in the course of carrying out activities with clients and to stay within their legally and professionally defined domains of practice. By doing so in their screening of clients, in their delivery of service, and in their provision of advice and recommendations, they can enhance their delivery of service while reducing the risks of claim and suit.

Date _____ Location _____

Subject _____ Persons or company involved _____

Comments:

Signed _____ Date _____

This form may be used to document incidents involving discussions with individual athletes, as well as such actions as changing program protocols or modifying the facility or its equipment.

Figure 7.6 Sample documentation form.
From National Strength and Conditioning Association (1994).

Bibliography

American College of Sports Medicine (1991). *Guidelines for exercise testing and prescription* (4th ed.). Philadelphia: Lea & Febiger.

American College of Sports Medicine (1992). *Health and fitness facility standards and guidelines.* Champaign, IL: Human Kinetics.

DeRouren v Holiday Spa Health Clubs of California, No. 346987, Superior Court of Los Angeles, CA (1988).

Herbert, D. (1987). Is there a legally mandated duty to screen exercise participants prior to exercise? *The Exercise Standards and Malpractice Reporter,* **1**(1), 10-12.

Herbert, D. (1988a). Are GXTs required for screening of all men over 40? *The Exercise Standards and Malpractice Reporter,* **2**(2), 18.

Herbert, D. (1988b). An examination of four recent cases against fitness instructors. *The Exercise Standards and Malpractice Reporter,* **2**(3), 45-47.

Herbert, D. (1989). Failure to warn/correct judged: Willful-wanton. *Fitness Management Magazine.*

Herbert, D. (1992). New litigation: Exercise without GXT results in defense verdict. *The Exercise Standards and Malpractice Reporter,* **5**(6), 90-92.

Herbert, D. (1993). Trainer and coach liable for non-referral of student/athlete to physician. *The Exercise Standards and Malpractice Reporter,* **7**(1), 12-13.

Herbert, D., & Herbert, W. (1993). *Legal aspects of preventive, rehabilitative and recreational exercise programs* (3rd ed.). Canton, OH: Professional Reports.

Koeberle, B. (1990). *Legal aspects of personal fitness training.* Canton, OH: Professional Reports.

National Strength and Conditioning Association. (1994). *Essentials of strength training and conditioning.* Champaign, IL: Human Kinetics.

State v Winterich, 157 Ohio St. 414 (1952).

Stetina v State Medical Licensing Board, 513 N.E. 2nd 1234, Indiana App. 2 District (1987).

Part III

The *Personal* Part of Personal Training

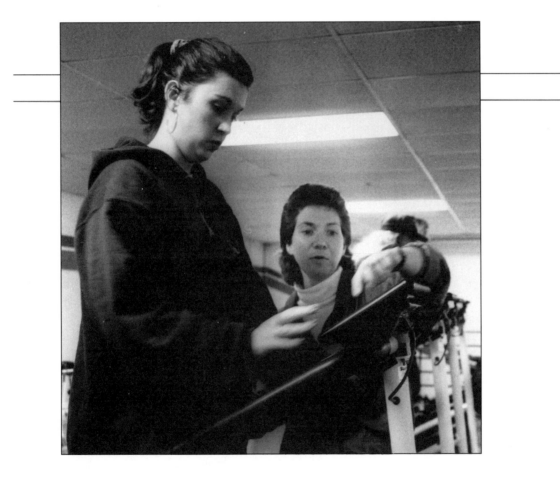

Part III of this book focuses in on the *personal* side of personal training. As the title suggests, personal trainers are involved in a profession in which there is high degree of personal contact with people. An aerobics instructor has to feel comfortable in front of a group of people, whereas a personal trainer has to feel comfortable in a one-on-one situation. As previously discussed, personal trainers wear many hats. This section discusses techniques that help personal trainers function while wearing all those different hats.

This section begins with a chapter written by two highly respected personal trainers, Kathy Alexander and Irv Rubenstein. Although knowledge of business, exercise, and nutrition is important to personal trainers, if you don't know how to communicate with your clients, you won't last long in the business! Chapter 8 presents essential information on the unique relationship between a client and a personal trainer. It explains why it is important to understand both the personal trainer's and client's responsibilities. Once the ground rules have been outlined, training can start. When clear and concise rules are not discussed before establishing a relationship, conflict often arises. Often clients think personal trainers are there just to serve their needs, and only their needs. When clients show up late, or cancel appointments several minutes before a session is about to start, you need to let them know that your time is just as valuable as theirs; any client who doesn't agree with you needs to find another trainer! This chapter defines the client–trainer relationship and discusses ways to strengthen it. Understanding the client–trainer relationship is essential for success as a personal trainer.

Chapter 9 looks at the psychology of personal training. James and Nettie Gavin present a simple and effective model to help personal trainers communicate more effectively, to help the trainer and client better understand each others' needs, and to help foster a relationship that meets everyone's needs. The chapter presents essential information on the psychology of personal training and outlines the SPIRIT model of one-on-one relationships.

Chapter 10, written by Jack Jones, presents essential information on how to work effectively with clients by improving your teaching and communication techniques. You might have a PhD in exercise or nutrition, but if you don't know how to teach effectively, you won't be able to share your knowledge. A primary function of all personal trainers is to teach—teach clients how to perform a particular exercise, how to stay motivated, or how to lose weight. Jones provides teaching techniques for personal trainers.

Finally, chapter 11, written by Douglas Brooks, presents essential information on the art and science of program design. The scientific part is usually the easy part. The art of program design is the challenging part. How do you design the most effective and appropriate exercise program for someone? One way is by listening carefully to the needs of the individual. The initial client interview helps you obtain necessary information to plan a safe and effective exercise program, based on the needs of individual clients. With time, trainers learn to develop more creative exercise programs. Chapter 11 also reviews important procedures that need to be followed before starting someone on an exercise program and concludes with some great ways to make exercise programs more creative and effective.

Chapter 8

The Client–Trainer Relationship

Kathy Alexander
Irv Rubenstein

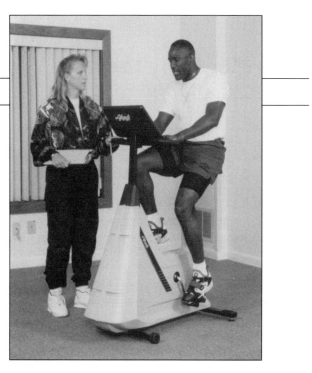

The objectives of this chapter are to

- discuss the unique relationship between a personal trainer and a client,
- consider various client profiles, and
- discuss the mechanics of the business relationship.

Overview

You can be a great businessperson and a very knowledgeable personal trainer, but if you don't know how to communicate with your clients, you won't last long in the business! This chapter presents essential information on the unique relationship between a client and a personal trainer. Some trainers may have never given the topic a great deal of consideration, but they should. It is important to understand the division of responsibilities between the personal trainer and the client. The trainer and client should openly discuss their mutual responsibilities prior to starting the training process. If the separate roles are not discussed, conflict may arise later. This chapter defines the client–trainer relationship and discusses ways to strengthen it. Understanding the client–trainer relationship is essential for success as a personal trainer.

The one-to-one relationship that personal trainers have with their clients presents a unique opportunity to positively influence the lifestyle and environment of another person. The broad and various benefits of personal training are accomplished through effecting changes in the client's lifestyle. Personal trainers need to understand that their role in the relationship, both as trainer and as professional businessperson, contributes to the client's willingness and ability to effect lifestyle changes, such as increasing fitness, stopping smoking, or managing stress. This chapter describes the various roles of a personal trainer and the various types of clients they are likely to encounter.

Roles Played by the Personal Trainer

In order to be successful, today's personal trainer must have both formal and technical training and skills in a variety of areas. A good personal trainer is an educator, motivator, and manager. Once personal trainers develop a relationship with a client, they must work hard at keeping the client. As you read through this chapter, think about your strong and weak points when it comes to the client–trainer relationship. Develop a plan of action that will improve your weak areas.

Educator

One of the most important roles that a trainer plays is that of educator. This role requires the trainer to elicit as clear a statement of goals as possible from the client, to reiterate these in light of physiological and biomechanical realities, and then restate them. After assisting the client in setting reasonable goals, the trainer should dedicate a portion of the first few training sessions to educating the client on specific exercises and activities that will allow them to achieve their fitness and performance goals. This often requires the trainer to add or eliminate equipment or activities based on orthopaedic or health limitations. Each session of supervised exercise should also emphasize proper form and breathing techniques.

The trainer should describe the proposed fitness plan. This discussion provides a perfect opportunity to teach basic anatomy and exercise physiology concepts as they relate to the client's goals, as well as to note a client's physical or health concerns. Most clients possess some amount of outdated or inaccurate information that needs to be updated. It has

been the experience of the authors that the more clients understand the scientific concepts behind an exercise program, the more likely they are to follow the program. It is during this educational process that the trainer really begins to earn his or her position of authority and trust with the client.

Additional areas of instruction include calculation of exercise-training heart rate, as well as proper technique for accurate heart rate monitoring. The inclusion of the Borg scale of ratings of perceived exertion (see Figure 8.1) along with or instead of direct heart rate monitoring can be another way to monitor exercise intensity. Some clients, particularly those who require more specific monitoring or those who like electronic gadgetry, may want to purchase and use an electronic digital heart rate monitor.

Personal trainers must continue to educate themselves also by reading journal articles, books, and newsletters and joining professional organizations

6	No exertion at all
7	Extremely light
8	
9	Very light
10	
11	Light
12	
13	Somewhat hard
14	
15	Hard (heavy)
16	
17	Very hard
18	
19	Extremely hard
20	Maximal exertion

Figure 8.1 The Borg ratings of perceived exertion (RPE) scale.
Reprinted from Borg (1985).

such as American College of Sports Medicine, American Council on Exercise, the International Association of Fitness Professionals, and the National Strength and Conditioning Association. Read the publications that these organizations produce and attend their continuing education seminars. You will learn how to update clients' exercise programs to reflect the most current information in personal training and exercise science, helping both you and your clients stay enthusiastic during the training process.

Motivator

Another primary role of the trainer is to motivate the client to stay involved in the exercise process long enough to experience benefits and reach goals. Often this requires the trainer to urge clients to push beyond their usual comfort zones. Many clients will do the last 1 to 2 repetitions on a weight machine only with the encouragment of their trainer.

Some clients may want a personal trainer to perform a fitness assessment and design a workout program for them to execute on their own. The trainer might then consider giving the client only a portion of the workout program at a time. For instance, a trainer can design and demonstrate the upper-body–strength workout and tell the client to do the routine four times before returning for the next session. Typically the client returns with some questions and may indicate if any of the activities are uncomfortable or painful. After reviewing and correcting this portion of the program, the trainer would give the next portion of the workout. This process allows the client to ease into the program. We recommend holding 3-5 sessions with specific goals and careful monitoring, followed by sessions at a mutually agreeable frequency. Be sure to schedule the next appointment before the client leaves. If the client agrees to a monthly or quarterly follow-up session, review and update the workout routine in order to maximize fitness and health benefits, as well as to keep the client motivated.

Manager

An often forgotten and neglected area of personal training is client follow-up. It is important to refer to the client's original goals periodically and to make sure that the exercise program is consistent with the stated goals and any fitness assessment results that are available. Goals should be updated periodically and appropriate adjustments made to the exercise program. Often clients will do some portion of their weekly workouts on their own. It is not unusual for

a client to train with a trainer for one to three sessions and work out on their own several times a week. It is critical that the trainer make specific recommendations, such as to jog 30 minutes twice a week, perform a weight routine once a week, and attend two workout sessions with the trainer. The trainer should ask for a specific recall of the client's activity between workout sessions. Quickly the clients learn that they are in fact involved in a process that is being monitored, and this knowledge typically increases the likelihood that they will continue to work out alone. Independent workouts and activities are an important part of a client's total fitness program, as well as an important ingredient in eventually becoming independent of the trainer.

Once the client demonstrates a basic understanding of fitness principles and indicates a desire to become more independent, set up an appointment for the follow-up visit. Remind clients that you are available by phone if they have a question. (Note: Questions that can't be answered in 3-5 minutes should be dealt with one-on-one in a paid training session.) Some trainers do allow phone consultations that last longer than 5 minutes. If this is part of your service, then advertise it and discuss this policy in the initial visit. For the few clients who don't want to schedule a follow-up appointment or can't afford to do so, it is important that the trainer still maintain phone call follow-up.

As the trainer–client relationship grows, it is not unusual for clients to share more and more of their personal lives. Trainers who work with clients over a period of months and years will find themselves sharing their clients' job changes, marriages, births of children, divorces, deaths of loved ones, new homes, etc. The client is best served by the trainer who listens in a nonjudgmental way and maintains client confidentiality. Most clients really just enjoy the opportunity to express themsleves and don't expect any more than an empathetic ear. However, if a client asks for advice that is beyond the scope of personal training, the trainer may need to refer the client to a community service organization. While your relationship with a client might develop into a friendship, you must maintain a professional distance in order to properly manage the client's program.

Client Profiles

Each client is an individual with a distinct history and perception of both the world and the self. Likewise, each client seeks the advice and assistance of a trainer for distinct reasons (despite the groupings we will be making below). That is, while Client A and Client B may both seek to lose 10 pounds, their reasons, goals, and methods must be considered individually. When trainers recognize individual differences and needs, they become true *personal* trainers.

In our combined years of training and consulting, we have identified five basic types of clients. These groupings are not mutually exclusive; often a client fits into two or more categories. These personality types are the Improvers, the Adapters, the Preemptors, the Rehabbers, and the Achievers.

The Improver

The Improver seeks to make small gains in general fitness that may include reducing body fat or gross weight, often for cosmetic purposes. Sometimes the improver already eats and exercises appropriately but needs professional advice or stimulus to get those last few pounds or inches off. It is not uncommon to find structural or functional imbalances in strength due to lifestyle or sport activities that need fine tuning. Improvers seek to prepare for the continued stresses and strains brought on by habitual activity, posture, or by age alone. The Improver may need a boost in intensity, additional exercises for the lower back, shoulder external rotators, or simply some specific flexibility exercises. The Improver may see the trainer once a week or less frequently. This type of client benefits from regular follow-ups, either through phone calls or visits.

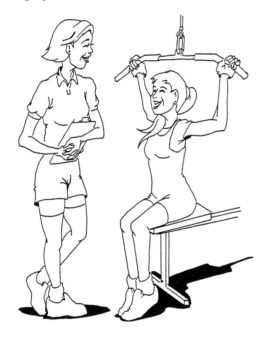

The Adapter

The Adapter, not unlike the Improver, is trying to improve healthy lifestyle components. Adapters are striving to improve fitness parameters, such as aerobic capacity, body fatness, strength, or flexibility by initiating an exercise program under the guidance and supervision of a professional. The Adapter may not be a regular exerciser, may be a formerly active athlete or exerciser on a very long sabbatical due to schooling, family, or professional obligations, or may have been advised by a health care professional to begin exercising. It is not uncommon for members of this group to be trying to reduce their weight significantly enough to lower blood pressure, cholesterol level, and other cardiac risk factors. This type of client may require more gentle motivation; the trainer needs to be cautious about overstraining, overeducating, and understimulating the Adapter.

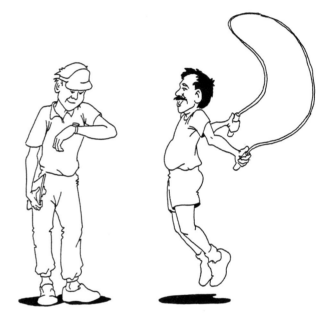

Boredom, fear of failure, pain, or discomfort—these probably have inhibited the Adapter's past attempts at exercising and training. Self-consciousness about body shape and coordination may be a big factor. These clients may do best when the gym is least crowded, or in a home setting. However, there are multiple benefits from getting the client comfortable with the gym setting, especially from the standpoint of lifestyle adaptation (accessibility and cost) and self-esteem. Adapters need the I-can-do-it approach to life because many years of inactivity, illness, disease, or injury may have also scarred their self-image.

The Preemptor

The Preemptor is a combination of the Improver and the Adapter. The subtle difference is often in the degree of improvement needed in the basic fitness parameters and the degree of psychological considerations the trainer initially must take into account. The Preemptor seeks to "get healthy." Preemptors want to be able to play ball with their children, to live a more fruitful and energetic life, if not a longer one; to start eating properly; to improve their physical condition above their current status of normal or average; and to ensure a less painful or disabled future.

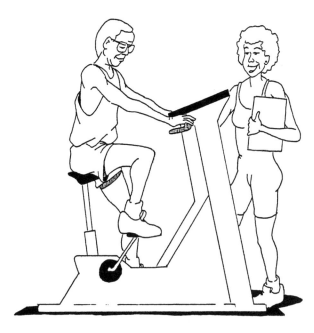

The Preemptor is basically healthy and perhaps older, late 40s to mid-70s, and chooses exercise before medical advice is needed. Sometimes, the younger Preemptor simply wants to maintain current levels of fitness and health; training is a means to an end. Preemptors want to train efficiently, properly, and maybe even enjoyably; they are preparing for the future by seeking an experienced and knowledgeable trainer.

In working with Preemptors, as with Adapters, trainers need to offer information and strategies that will fit easily into their lifestyles. For the Preemptor, like the Improver, the information should be both physically and emotionally stimulating. Finally, the emphasis should not be on increasing intensity and duration; rather, Preemptors often work better with increased frequency, even without the trainer, if the other two components are minimized.

The Rehabber

The Rehabber arrives with an injury and presents a different challenge each time, even when the injury is one the trainer has seen previously. First of all, most trainers are not physical therapists. Recognizing

and acknowledging this fact will prevent both misrepresentation and possible litigation. However, a trainer should have working knowledge of anatomy, kinesiology, and biomechanics to be capable of adapting standard training techniques to the injured "athlete." Thus, the trainer should provide a workout that conditions the injured area(s) without aggravating it (them). Simultaneously, because therapists and even doctors tend to ignore other components of fitness if a patient has a specific injury (unless the patient is an elite athlete), the trainer must consider the whole person, not just the injured area. Sometimes the injury prevents continuation of the client's previous program; often it hampers recreational activity; occasionally it interferes with work. It is the trainer's goal to teach proper body mechanics and posture and to condition the cardiovascular system, in addition to strengthening and stretching the injured muscles.

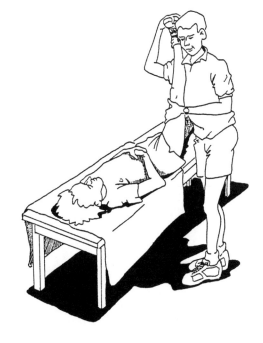

The Achiever

The Achiever is the competitive athlete. Competition doesn't necessarily imply other participants. It may refer to his or her own fitness data, such as run times or distance, weight lifted, muscle size, or tone. Achievers are often fun to train because they will follow your advice. However, their demands are occasionally out of professional bounds, and it may be necessary for you to take control of a situation and perhaps even terminate it. For example, young female athletes often get caught up in the "female athlete triad"—disordered eating, amenorrhea, osteoporosis—and seek a trainer who can help them succeed in their fitness or athletic endeavors. These clients sometimes don't want to listen to reason based on scientific fact. Another common example is the willingness of competitors to use experimental training or nutritional techniques or aids that may be inappropriate for specific individuals or even contraindicated for anyone until more research is available. It may become necessary to send the client elsewhere for help (e.g., a sport psychologist, nutritionist, orthopaedist, etc.). It is our firm belief that trainers must follow principles based on the best medical and legal information. So, while the Achiever may be fun to train, the over-Achiever may try to compromise your professionalism. Remember, *you*, as a professional, must control the relationship.

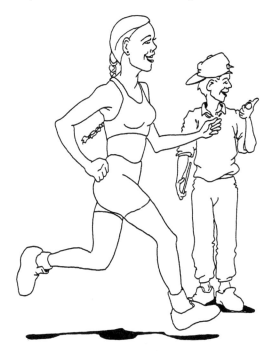

The Nature of the Relationship

The general components of the client–trainer relationship are not unlike the guidelines established by the Ten Commandments: broad principles with lots of room for personal and professional interpretation. In this section we will discuss the parameters of professional behavior and the atmosphere of the personal training setting. It is not our intention to define specific and concrete rules because a professional trainer must tailor programs according to the type of client and the training setting. It is our contention that the client–trainer relationship depends entirely on the amount and quality of trust the client places

in the trainer. Without trust, your advice, knowledge, and coaching are useless.

Professionalism

Professional decorum is the pathway to establishing trust. The initial contact with a client may take place on the phone, in person, or even through a mediator such as a physician or therapist. The client's first impression of you sets the tone for the relationship. Trainers must establish themselves as professionals in demeanor, knowledge, and appearance; appropriate use of language and active listening skills are essential.

While one of the benefits of this profession is the freedom to wear comfortable athletic clothing and shoes, your clothing should always be clean, in good repair, and appropriate to the client and setting. A trainer who wears a minimal bikini or thong leotards looks less than professional, possibly even threatening or offensive.

Clarity

While it is important to remember that the client's needs and interests always take precedence, it is the trainer's responsibility to establish and maintain the boundaries of the relationship. We refer to this as *clarity*. In the initial meeting it is important to clarify your specific policies on appointment setting, cancellations, fees, and means of communication (telephone, beeper, answering machine, etc.). It is also valuable to agree in advance to discuss any discomfort or dissatisfaction on either the client's or trainer's part. At some point in the early stages of the relationship, the trainer must assert authority and leadership without appearing arrogant. A trainer must be an active listener without appearing judgmental, an educator without being an evangelist, a service provider without being an accommodator. That is, while acknowledging that the client (like the customer) is always right, the trainer must render services that are scientifically and legally supportable. If the client wants to lose 20 pounds in 40 days, and the trainer agrees that this desire is reasonable, the trainer must guide and direct the client towards proper and correct exercise and nutritional behaviors. Clarity is the foundation for the trust that must develop for success in the relationship and program.

Confidentiality

Another cornerstone of trust is the medicolegal assurance of *confidentiality*, the breach of which may have legal ramifications for privacy violations, and the social standard of discretion. The client must have confidence that all medical, psychological, personal, and other private matters discussed or written (on intake forms) will be handled professionally. Thus, not only should documents be maintained in order, they should be kept in a safe and exclusive setting, inaccessible to other professionals or clients. Likewise, the information a client shares with the trainer should remain private. Of course, discretion is an open-ended mandate; sometimes one client's experiences can provide a general lesson for another. However, avoid using names or other identifying data in such conversations. You must always maintain the anonymity of your clients—even at staff meetings or professional gatherings where people discuss case histories. Generalities may be discussed where relevant. Personal, social, employment, and other identifying information must be held in confidence because clients often reveal sensitive information about themselves in the personal training setting, information that could damage their standing in the community if it became public, and thus expose the trainer to liability.

A Safe Haven

Professional decorum, clarity, and confidentiality create the setting for personal training as a safe haven for the client. By *safe haven* we mean a place and a relationship in which clients can be themselves, unjudged, unfettered, uninhibited. Of course, this does not permit criminal or sociopathic behavior, but it does allow clients to use profanities if they choose, to wear tattered exercise clothes, or to discuss personal issues without feeling threatened by the trainer's moral judgment. Freedom allows clients to divulge the dysfunctional or compulsive behaviors for which they may be seeking help. This information may assist the trainer in both continuing the training process and making appropriate referrals to adjunct professionals.

Occasionally a trainer may work with an offensive client. While trying to maintain the safe haven concept, the trainer should make a clear statement (or a discreet suggestion) that inappropriate or offensive behavior won't be tolerated. The risk of losing a client is present, but the risk of passive-aggressive behavior on the trainer's part is much more costly.

Open to Experimentation

Another aspect of the trust relationship is the willingness and the ability to *experiment* with and experience new health and exercise habits. This is readily

apparent when the client exhibits self-destructive behavior such as overeating or overexercising. Without trust, your recommended alternatives and adaptations will go unheeded. Always consider the client's interests, no matter what you propose. In other words, do not push your agenda on the client, but create an atmosphere in which you affirm your client's agenda.

Friendship

The client–trainer relationship often becomes very intimate. The frequency and privacy of sessions encourages the client to treat the trainer as confidant and friend. For the bi- or triweekly client, the 1-hour sessions may amount to the most private time a client has with any one individual; training sessions may become treasured moments in the week when the client is at the center of another's attention. In fact, for some clients it is a time not to think, but to be told what to do and simply do it. The most high-powered executives, it seems, succumb to the role of student, slave, or athlete. The friendship that develops in the gym occasionally spills out into restaurants, movies, or homes. Whether clients and trainers are the same or opposite gender, married or single, this new aspect of the relationship may complicate the training relationship.

Another difficult situation that may arise is when clients or trainers use the relationship to further their own business contacts or agendas. This crossover into a second business relationship, outside the training environment, may strain the trust relationship and interfere with the client's original training goals and intentions. Often training is a time for clients to nurture their overall health, emotional and physical, and the introduction of a business proposition will alter that experience. Much like the adage regarding family, never mix business with clients.

Generosity

Generosity is the final component of the client–trainer relationship. This is not a gift-giving concept. Rather, generosity deals with the natural leniency you might offer a client. For instance, while you do depend on a client for your income, you may decide to be more lenient in accepting sudden scheduling changes for a client whose job hours are erratic. Another example of generosity is how you implement a rate increase. One trainer, for example, might split the difference between current and future rates with long-time clients. Another may offer a time frame to permit transition to the new fee structure.

Others may suggest a more vigorous nontrainer program for a client, with less frequent but still regular training sessions.

Whatever you do, operate with the client in mind. This reassures clients that your interest in them is more than monetary and reaffirms that their success is what both of you consider important. Thus, you can make a living and career out of helping people help themselves get, be, and stay healthy and fit.

Mechanics of the Business Relationship

The purpose of this section is to help readers create a professional persona with clients and other professionals in order to perform at the highest caliber, as well as to promote themselves and their services. The mechanics of doing business are the initial contact (business cards and telephone), appointment setting (including missed and late appointments), office environment, fees, extra services and charges, rate increases and changes, ethics, and self-promotion.

Interacting With Clients

The initial contact is obviously your potential client's first opportunity to assess you as a knowledgeable and professional provider of a unique service. Whether this contact occurs in person, over the phone, or by the exchange of business cards, you are being judged on how you present yourself. Regardless of the quality of your physique, your professional demeanor will determine your success not just with that client but with the entire pool of potential clients. In your first presentation you need to be able to say who you are and what you do in a concise, nonthreatening manner.

Face-to-face initial contacts may occur anywhere—in the gym, at a party, or in another place of business. You need to be able to discuss your profession without appearing to be drumming up business. You need to direct the conversation so that you give basic information, not consultation, and explain how you operate your business. Your business card should state your services, your qualifications, and phone numbers. (For a trainer without access to an office setting, in or out of a gym, you may wish to consider having a mailing address other than your home, a post office box, for example, or not including an address at all). Similarly, your telephone message should reflect the same attributes as your card and your in-person presentation in tone and in content. Basically, your goals during this initial contact are to market yourself, invite the person to consider becoming a client, establish the tone of the business relationship, and represent the profession of personal training in a positive light.

Setting the appointment is typically the next step in the process. While it may seem very simple to designate a time and place, there are three points to consider. First, orally, in writing (on an appointment card), or both, repeat the time, date, place, and the cost of the appointment. Second, restate the nature of the meeting, what the client can expect, what to eat and drink before training, and what to wear. Third, reiterate the conditions of late appointments and cancellations and indicate how you can be reached. These considerations demonstrate the nature of communication and the level of professionalism the client can expect from you.

An important aspect of professionalism is the trainer's office. The designation of *office* goes beyond a desk and chair. The office is any space other than the actual training or gym floor from which trainers conduct other aspects of their business. For example, this is a quieter, more private space suitable for fitness testing, exercise feedback and prescription, nutrition and diet, goal setting, and discussions of personal issues. Also, this is where you arrange appointments, discuss and exchange fees, and maintain records and files. Even if you do not have a private room, a quiet corner and a briefcase can, with a little creativity, create an office in any training setting.

Setting Business Policies

Any discussion about fees and rates is sensitive. However, the manner in which you handle this will contribute to the tone of the entire relationship. You want to present your fees in a straightforward way as your fee structure represents the value of the services you provide. It is best to be very clear about your fees and when you expect to be paid, be it on an appointment basis, weekly, or monthly. State your policies on billing, record keeping, cancellations, late appointments, partial sessions, etc.

In discussing your fees, include a statement regarding special services and their costs. For example, fitness testing, nutritional counseling (if you are qualified to do so), off-site training, alternative trainings (e.g., road races, mountain bike excursions, in-line skating) are some services you may offer that require a different fee structure. Additionally, if you have been in the profession long enough to have gained valuable experience and extra education and certification, a time may come when your fees need to reflect these changes. Rate increases need to be presented in a manner as professional as the initial setting of fees. You may feel more comfortable if you explain the reasons for the rate increase, such as recently obtained degrees or certifications. While doing so, provide a face-saving opening or option that permits the client to continue the training process, either with you on a less frequent basis or with another trainer whom you could recommend.

While our experience has been that most clients rarely alter their training schedules because of a rate increase, in the unlikely event that the client does change trainers, you should maintain an open-door policy if the client later chooses to return. (Of course, your new fee would be in force.) Finally, there may be certain clients for whom a rate increase may be a deterrent and, for whatever reasons, you may choose not to impose the increase. However, it is important to discuss this with the individual clients, letting them know that this is a confidential, private agreement between the two of you.

During the initial session(s), it is necessary to establish some boundaries around your personal and professional lives. Thus, it is at this time that you specify where and when you can be reached for routine matters, when and how you may be reached in emergencies, and any extra charges for phone consultations or emergency visits. For example, some professionals charge a dollar per minute for calls lasting more than 5 minutes. You may also wish to specify the items and days of your availability to train and your policies regarding weekends and holidays. Again, clarity, honesty, and consistency remain the foundations of your professional relationship with the client and will continue to provide the structure of the client's ongoing fitness process.

Maintaining Professional Conduct

The ethical considerations for a personal trainer are not unlike those for anyone else in the helping professions. Some of these we have already discussed: confidentiality, respect of boundaries, clarity, and honesty, as well as the transition from a business relationship to one that includes friendship. One area which has yet to receive much attention is that of physical contact, or touch. The very nature of personal training includes a large measure of touch, whether it be in spotting, correcting technique or posture, or doing assisted flexibility exercises. We call this appropriate touch and distinguish it from sensual or sexual touch. Each client comes in with a distinct background, agenda, and comfort level about physical contact. Thus you may encounter a variety of responses to touch. It is not uncommon for a client to choose to work with a particular trainer based on an agenda centered around the necessity of physical contact. For example, one woman may prefer being stretched by another female whereas another may choose to be stretched by a male. The comfort or discomfort one might feel and derive from this type of contact may be a contributing factor in the success of that client's overall process.

Marketing Yourself

The final consideration for a professional in a service-oriented business is that your best advertisement is the success of your clients. The manner in which you conduct your business and apply the sport science principles will determine both the satisfaction your clients receive from the experience and their enthusiasm for sharing that experience with those around them. However, it is not inappropriate to ask for business. For example, you might offer to speak at certain functions or groups in which your clients are involved, and never hesitate to ask for referrals. In other words, it is absolutely appropriate to market yourself in a discreet and professional manner.

Summary

The client–trainer relationship has all the complexities of any other relationship. As a member of a helping profession, you are entrusted with your clients' personal well-being as well as their physical well-being. The potential for conflict is there, but so is the potential for success. Consider your commitment to the career of personal fitness training. What kind of a trainer do you want to be? Your answer will determine whether your relationships with clients will be mutually beneficial and profitable.

Suggested Readings

Brammer, L.M. (1973). *The helping relationship.* Englewood Cliffs, NJ: Prentice-Hall.

Combs, A.W., & Avila, D.L. (1985). *Helping relationships: Basic concepts for the helping professions* (3rd ed.). Boston: Allyn and Bacon.

Rogers, C. (1961). *On becoming a person.* Boston: Houghton Mifflin.

Whitmyer, C., Rasberry, S., & Phillips, S. (1989). *Running a one-person business.* Berkeley, CA: Ten Speed Press.

Chapter 9

The Psychology of Personal Training

James Gavin
Nettie Gavin

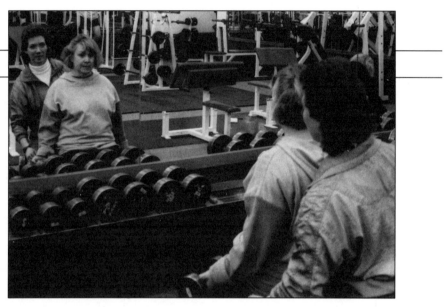

The objectives of this chapter are to

- identify core psychological principles for personal training through the SPIRIT model;
- increase personal trainers' awareness of psychological issues in working with others; and
- demonstrate ways of creating the essential conditions for effective relationships with clients.

Overview

Psychology is the science of human behavior. Its principles are important to the field of personal training because they can help trainers understand themselves, their clients, and the needs each brings to their relationship. This chapter represents a creative integration of essential principles of psychology as they relate to one-to-one relationships. At the core of this chapter is the SPIRIT model of relationship dynamics. (For a deeper exploration of the SPIRIT model, see *Psychology for Health Fitness Professionals* by James and Nettie Gavin, 1995, Human Kinetics.) Integrating the SPIRIT principles will help you realize your full potential as a personal trainer.

What is the essence of effective human relationships? How can you give people exactly what they need to do their best and, at the same time, keep yourself in top psychological shape? This chapter describes a psychology of interpersonal relationships captured in the word SPIRIT—the one you have and the one you want to share with others. The word will be the magic in your work. It will reveal your path to success. It will give you the winning edge in a game where there are no losers, and it will enhance all dimensions of your life.

The SPIRIT Model

Health and fitness are about the whole person, not just the body and not just the mind. We know the whole person incorporates something more—a special ingredient mostly known through extraordinary moments: persistence toward seemingly unreachable goals, transformations in life direction, and simple acts of profound courage.

However, this special ingredient can be present in all moments of life, not just extraordinary ones. We would like to show you how to incorporate SPIRIT into your work, into your training relationships, and into your connection with yourself. Each letter of the word SPIRIT has a special meaning (see Figure 9.1):

S — Support

P — Purpose

I — Integrity

R — Resolving conflict

I — Inspiration

T — Timing

"You must be Lulu Ryder," Hank said as he greeted his new client. "Before we begin working together, I'd like to hear why you decided to hire a personal trainer," Hank continued as Lulu made herself comfortable.

Lulu paused reflectively and then spoke. "I've tried to exercise regularly in the past, but I just can't stay with a routine. I've come to realize that to stick with it I need some support."

Hank smiled easily and asked, "Lulu, how do you see me providing that support?"

SUPPORT: Support involves a willingness to hear your client with empathy, caring, and fairness. It's being responsible to yourself as you stand by your client in his or her quest for wholeness.

PURPOSE: Toward what end or purpose will you support your client? Your purpose is framed by three questions: What is your role? What are your resources? What is the situation?

INTEGRITY: Integrity is founded on self-respect and an ethical stance that acknowledges your humanity. It extends to your client through clear agreements that are jointly determined and honored.

RESOLVING CONFLICTS: Resolving conflicts involves facing what doesn't feel "right" in one-to-one relationships. It requires separating emotions from facts, and working toward win-win solutions based on fairness and respect.

INSPIRATION: Inspiration is encouraging clients to find the place inside that feels like "home." It comes from a deep place of self-acceptance and speaking from your heart.

TIMING: Timing is knowing when to intervene—when to listen and when to ask the next question; when to suggest change and when to reestablish boundaries; when to confront and when to say good-bye; when to be there for your client and when to be there for yourself.

Figure 9.1 The SPIRIT model of relationships.

"That's a good question, Hank. I think I know why I always quit before. It was probably because I thought there was something wrong with me that needed to be fixed. So, what I mostly need from you is encouragement and agreement that I don't need to look like the cover of any fitness magazine."

Hank surveyed this middle-aged, heavy-set woman with tired-looking eyes. He knew that most clients said something about wanting to lose weight or shape up within the first 5 minutes of meeting him, yet he sensed this woman's agenda was different. How could he help her explore her motives?

He ventured a question. "You don't want me to tell you I'm going to make you look like a fitness ad, so what do you want? And how can I best support your intentions?"

Lulu realized she had not told the whole story. "Hank, this may sound a bit blunt, but I don't want to feel pushed by your need to feel successful. I've been operating on that strategy too long and without much success. Sure, I want to lose weight and get in shape, but not at the cost of my self-esteem. I have a great job, but it's stressful, and I need this time to be enjoyable. If I start placing all kinds of expectations for change on this program, I know I'll just quit again."

Hank wanted to make sure he was getting the right picture. He said, "Lulu, you want to work with me on a program that is enjoyable and that helps you relieve stress. You want to work toward losing weight and getting fit, but you don't want to go about it as if it were a crisis or as if there were something wrong with you." Hank paused before asking, "Is that it?"

Now, it was Lulu's turn to smile. "Hank, that's exactly what I mean. As I was rehearsing my reasons for coming to see you today, I was trying to figure out whether I should tell you I wanted to lose 20 or 25 pounds—all the while hearing part of me getting mad for not liking myself the way I am!"

Support

If we asked a hundred people what support looks like we could expect as many answers. So often we try to support others in ways that feel good to us, yet these may be the very ways that turn others off. When we first meet clients, it's critical to learn what they need—and how they see us helping them reach their goals. The temptation to jump in with ideas, plans, and an enthusiastic promise of success can backfire if we don't probe and listen for answers that may contradict our initial impressions.

Support doesn't always mean propping up another person or playing leader to their follower. More likely, it involves listening to them with fresh ears, and a willingness to acknowledge their concerns with empathy and respect. Listening is an art, and art takes practice. The more we listen, the more we hear how we can help.

When a client says, "I just want to learn to relax," and you can see that this person needs to lose weight, whose agenda do you follow? Do you try to convince the client that aerobic workouts produce profound states of relaxation? Or do you explore what relaxing exercise looks like to this person, and how you can best support this individual's needs?

After you learn who your client is, support translates into listening and acting in ways appropriate to your role as personal trainer and in ways that don't jeopardize your own values and needs. The most important skills for being supportive involve the willingness to hear another person without passing judgment; and without responding as the expert who really knows what is best for them.

Another way of understanding support is by considering what it is not. Support is not

- agreeing with whatever a person says;
- disagreeing because you know better;
- avoiding what a person says because it sounds difficult, ridiculous, or irrelevant;
- blaming the person for not following through or living up to commitments; or
- taking responsibility for achieving a person's goals.

Support is being as fully present as possible for your clients and putting your own agendas for them aside. It's allowing their goals to guide your work with them and measuring your success by their goals being met.

Purpose

Implicit in the definition of support is the concept of purpose. Toward what end or purpose are you supporting this client? Here is a formula to keep in mind when considering the concept of purpose. The formula has three words—role, resources, and situation—that frame your purpose in relation to that of your client. Ask yourself the following questions to clarify purpose.

- What is your role?
- What are your resources?
- What is the situation?

Role

The first question is about the nature of your job:

- What are you trained to do?
- What have you been hired to do?
- What are the legitimate tasks that you can perform?

If clients ask you to design a diet to accompany their training program, are you qualified to do so, and do you see this as part of your role? Is this how you are advertising yourself? Simply ask yourself, "Is this my job? Is this what I agreed to do?"

Resources

The second question is about your resources:

- What are your strengths and weaknesses in this moment?
- What options and facilities are available to you?
- Who else can you call on for assistance?

Are you tired and at your limit? Or do you have the energy to do what is requested of you, and still have sufficient resources to take care of your own needs?

Another aspect of resources deals with the possibility of delegating. Maybe someone else can handle the request or situation better, for example, a nutritionist for clients requesting diet information. It makes good sense to have a list of competent referral sources.

Also consider geographic resources: Where can you go and what can you do with your clients? Your resources may include the great outdoors or public swimming pools or rock climbing centers. If a client wants to learn to swim, find a pool.

Situation

The final consideration is the situation:

- What's happening right now in this situation?
- Is it a crisis?

Suppose your club manager wants you to take on another trainer's workload for a week while the trainer is on vacation. You could do it by adding three hours a day to your already full schedule. What do you do? Is this a crisis? Is your job at stake? Can the problem be solved another way?

Carol had a full day's work ahead of her: five clients, a class to teach, and her own workout. She was half out the door when the phone rang. It was Danny, her 10 a.m. client. He asked Carol to come to his house to train instead of meeting at the club. She did go to clients' homes, yet something didn't feel right, and she knew she had to say no.

"Danny, I want to stick to our original plan. I'll meet you at the club," she said deliberately.

"Why?" Danny asked with annoyance. "Why can't you come over here this morning?"

Carol responded carefully. "I would be willing to discuss this with you when we meet at the club. Right now I have to leave for an appointment."

Danny's emotions could be felt even before he spoke. "Well, Carol, maybe we just won't meet until you decide it's okay to train at my house."

Carol heard the threat. Danny trained three times a week, and reliable clients were in short supply. Yet, she knew her integrity was on the line. She responded evenly, "Danny, that's your decision. I'll be at the club at 10 a.m. as we originally agreed. Hope to see you then."

Ever since she had begun working with Danny, Carol felt a constant tension. Whether it was his style or his goal, Danny seemed intent on turning their one-to-one sessions into intimate encounters. No matter how strong and clear her messages were, the situation remained unchanged.

By 10:15 Carol decided Danny wasn't coming, but just then he sauntered out of the locker room.

"Bet you thought I wasn't going to show," Danny said coyly.

"You're right, Danny, I was just about to leave, but I'm really glad you're here. Would you like to have our discussion now or when we're finished working out?" Carol asked.

Danny seemed uncertain as he answered. "Well, how about we talk now and, if you're willing, we can train later?"

Carol opened the conversation. "Danny, it's important that I be clear about why I wouldn't go to your house. During the past 4 months, I let you know that your various attempts to get personal with me were not acceptable. Each time, you acknowledged your behavior, yet you continued with innuendoes, personal questions, and requests for dates. This morning, I felt the request to come to your house was a continuation of this agenda."

"Gee, Carol, I didn't know you were that serious. I'm sorry. I didn't realize how out of line I was," Danny said in earnest. "I want to keep working with you. You're a great trainer."

Integrity

Integrity is about ethics and boundaries. It's about fairness and respect, both toward yourself and your client. It's about clear agreements that you make and live by.

Carol's issue with Danny came from a sense that her personal integrity was being challenged. She had clear boundaries of appropriate behavior for herself and her clients, and Danny persistently tried to change them. When he made a request for her to train at his house, Carol's warning lights flashed. She felt she would be putting herself in a compromising situation, and giving Danny the reinforcement he needed to continue his chase.

It may be hard to take a stand, especially if your professional code of conduct is still evolving. Personal training is a relatively new profession. As such, professional codes of conduct may leave some gray areas. Even so, your personal code is more basic than your professional ones. How do you represent yourself? What are your values and beliefs? Figure 9.2 is a worksheet that may help you identify your professional boundaries.

An analysis of integrity is really a discussion about self and what you stand for. In all relationships, especially professional ones, letting others know your rules, limits, and boundaries is mandatory. Then, like a tennis court with its lines and boundaries, you get to call the action as fair or foul. You may know yourself well enough to clearly state your limits, rules, and boundaries in virtually any situation. Or you may struggle in some situations to figure out where you stand. On occasion, you may even find yourself saying one thing and doing another.

A trustworthy guide to personal integrity is, "If it doesn't feel right, respect your feelings enough to check it out." In the case of Carol and Danny, Carol felt that Danny had a hidden agenda and she trusted her gut feelings. It may have cost her a client, yet anything else might have been at the price of her self-esteem—not a very good trade. It's important to note here that Danny wasn't bad or wrong, but his behavior was inappropriate for Carol and the boundaries she set for professional relationships. The clearer your boundaries for time, money, style, and the personal side of training, the more comfortable and effective your working relationships will be.

Resolving Conflicts

A critical fact of conflict is that it occurs, whether we take an active role in it or not. Many times it seems

---

Write down your responses to the following statements:

"You should always . . ."

"You should never . . ."

"The way to be successful is to . . ."

"In working with my clients/athletes, it is my business to . . ."

"In working with my clients/athletes, it is none of my business to . . ."

"A good rule of thumb is . . ."

Figure 9.2 Statements to lead you to your boundaries. Reprinted from Gavin and Gavin (1995).

After you complete a conflict resolution meeting, use this checklist to determine whether you hit all the points or whether you left something out.

1.	Did you clarify to yourself what the conflict was about?	❏ Yes	❏ No
2.	Was it worth confronting?	❏ Yes	❏ No
3.	Did you arrange to confront the person at a good time and under favorable conditions?	❏ Yes	❏ No
4.	Did you factually describe the other person's actions?	❏ Yes	❏ No
5.	Did you indicate that the problem was of mutual concern?	❏ Yes	❏ No
6.	Did you define the conflict as specifically as possible?	❏ Yes	❏ No
7.	Did you accurately represent the effects of the conflict?	❏ Yes	❏ No
8.	Did you accurately present your emotional response to the conflict?	❏ Yes	❏ No
9.	Did you describe your part in the conflict—what you have done or omitted doing?	❏ Yes	❏ No
10.	Did you invite the other person to express her/his perceptions of the conflict?	❏ Yes	❏ No
11.	Did you verbally reflect your understanding of what the other person said to you?	❏ Yes	❏ No
12.	Did you generate potential solutions for mutual benefit with the other person's involvement?	❏ Yes	❏ No
13.	Did you work together in evaluating the potential solutions?	❏ Yes	❏ No
14.	Did you work out all the details of your mutual decision?	❏ Yes	❏ No
15.	Did you fully implement your solution?	❏ Yes	❏ No
16.	Did you set up a time and a place to discuss how the solution is working?	❏ Yes	❏ No

Figure 9.3   Checklist for resolving conflicts.
Reprinted from Gavin and Gavin (1995).

easier just to ignore conflict or smooth it over, hoping it will go away. Conflict is not a dirty word, yet it can become the arena where things get said and done that make or break relationships. Being able to sort out emotional reactions from the facts of situations will help you resolve areas of conflict or disagreement (see Figure 9.3).

One additional point about conflict is that your being right doesn't automatically make the other person wrong. Conflict may be frustrating or upsetting, but on a practical level all that it requires is that you deal with it. Effective conflict management may require asserting yourself again and again. It may even require that you change or end the relationship in order to maintain your personal integrity.

Self-respect and self-esteem are both the beginning and end points of conflict resolution. In the case of Carol and Danny, Carol realized Danny was trying to create a power struggle, yet she chose not to engage him in a manner that would undermine her integrity. She checked how she felt in the situation, decided what she needed in order to be okay both personally and professionally, then took her stand.

Inspiration

You don't have to believe in magic to realize that we all have the potential to deeply touch another person's life. We can do it without light shows or special gimmicks. Sometimes, it's as simple as allowing others to express themselves without our editing. When we encourage clients to be honest about their plans and exercise goals, we enable them to make a serious commitment.

Inspiration doesn't depend on pep talks or motivational magic. It comes from being yourself. Inspiration is living up to your agreements and holding your clients strictly accountable for their parts in the bargain. It means being honest, especially with yourself, and loving, also especially with yourself. Integrity and acceptance will be what your clients see when they look at you. What can be more inspirational than that?

Timing

Timing is knowing when to intervene: when to listen and when to ask the next question; when to suggest change and when to reestablish boundaries; when to confront and when to say good-bye; when to be there for others and when to be there for yourself. Developing this sense of the situation is not as hard as it sounds if you stay in touch with your feelings.

In the two scenarios we presented, timing was a critical element. Hank's interview with Lulu reflected timing in his choice of when to ask questions. Had Lulu shown resistance to his inquiries, he would have been cued that the time wasn't right for continuing the interview.

Carol sensed that it wasn't the right time to confront Danny on the phone. Carol's understanding of timing included the knowledge that it is not one sided; that is why she asked Danny if he preferred to talk before or after his training.

Being sensitive to the timing of words or actions will become central to your success.

Summary

We have approached the topic of psychology for personal trainers from the perspective of the self in relationships. Using the SPIRIT model as a guide to understanding both yourself and your clients will help you create the conditions necessary for successful one-to-one relationships. Each component of SPIRIT is of equal importance to the others. Think of them as a whole—like the word SPIRIT. Omit one letter and the whole is not the same. Keep them in mind like a fabric on which you work. See them in your actions, hear them in your words. Be them for your clients. Live them for yourself. May the SPIRIT be with you!

Suggested Reading

Gavin, J., & Gavin, N. (1995). *Psychology for health fitness professionals.* Champaign, IL: Human Kinetics.

Chapter 10

Working With Your Clients

Jack Jones

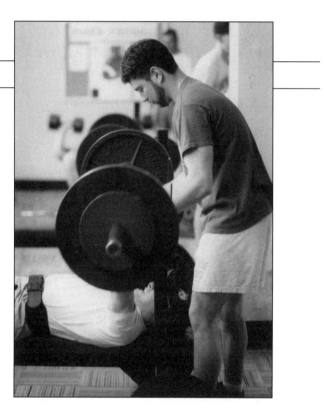

The objectives of this chapter are to

- discuss effective communication and teaching techniques,
- explain how to set short- and long-term goals, and
- suggest ways to motivate clients.

Overview

You can have a PhD in exercise or nutrition, but if you don't know how to teach effectively, you won't be able to share your knowledge. A primary function of all personal trainers is to teach: how to perform a particular exercise, how to stay motivated, or how to lose weight. Personal trainers can learn some simple teaching techniques to improve the way they communicate with their clients. This chapter presents essential information on how to improve your teaching and communication techniques.

An essential part of personal training is the ability to teach other people about fitness and nutrition. Do you know what kind of teacher you are? Most often people model their teaching styles after teachers they have had in the past. Ideally, you want to develop a teaching style that you are comfortable with. There are three basic requirements for effective teaching: a love for your subject, a desire to share it, and a basic competence in the subject.

The first two requirements are essential, and the third point is important, but not as important as the first two. The reason is that someone may be very knowledgeable about a particular subject, but will not be an effective teacher without the first two elements. You can always tell when someone loves to teach. You don't become a great teacher overnight; time and experience make a good teacher.

The process we call *teaching*—imparting knowledge from one person who knows more to others who know less—is complex. Teachers' techniques are as varied as teachers, because they evolve out of unique combinations of education, experience, and individual personality traits. But of all a teacher's techniques, communication by far is the most important. Whatever information the teacher is trying to convey, from English literature to weightlifting, the secret of conveying it successfully is knowing not only what, but how, to communicate.

Communication

We communicate to learn and acquire knowledge; to relate, establish, and maintain interpersonal relationships; to influence, control, manipulate, or direct others; to play, escape from work, and to enjoy life; and to help others. Communication can be very personal, such as communication with a loved one or close friend, or less personal, perhaps with a new client. Some people are good at communicating their thoughts to others, for example, a good public speaker, while others have trouble with simple communication, such as ordering a meal at a restaurant. The ability to communicate effectively can be improved by working on the nine communication skills described in Table 10.1.

For a personal trainer, understanding the benefits of specific exercise programs, which muscles ensure proper performance, and how to present this information to clients constitute technique. Explanation and demonstration involve communication. Of course, personal trainers communicate in many ways, not merely through words. The trainer's own body conditioning and grooming, his or her conduct

Table 10.1   Nine Behavioral Skills To Enhance Interpersonal Communication

1. Eye communication—Always make good eye contact. Nothing is more distracting than talking with someone who is looking down at your feet or up at the sky!
2. Posture—If standing, stand tall with your shoulders back. If sitting, sit up straight.
3. Body language—Learn to look relaxed. Avoid nervous gestures or exaggerated movements.
4. Appearance—Appearance can significantly improve your ability to communicate well. If you are trying to attract a new client, wear your best warm-up suit.
5. Voice—Speak clearly and use a commanding tone. A strong voice shows confidence.
6. Language—Excessive use of jargon, *O.K.*, pauses, etc. all reduce your communication abilities.
7. Listener involvement—Be a good listener. Take the time to listen clearly to the other person before responding.
8. Humor—Good humor is always helpful.
9. The natural self—Be yourself.

Adapted from Decker (1988).

in the club setting and outside, and a host of other factors are all part of communication.

How does a trainer project a professional image? Whenever trainers step onto the gym floor or talk to clients, they communicate with everyone within sight and earshot. Physical appearance is the trainer's first statement. You could be the best trainer in your town, but if you are 25-pounds overweight, your first statement is not a positive one. Your conditioning, clothes, and hair are all part of the image you communicate. Within the club setting, although uniforms are not a necessity, they do help communicate that personal trainers see themselves as professionals.

Another factor that precedes and facilitates contact with prospective clients is demeanor. A positive attitude, healthy self-confidence, general good health, and a pleasant way of relating to strangers are all evaluated quickly by anyone who sees you. Swaggering egotism communicates itself as well, though not positively. Probably the most lasting and realistic assessment of an individual is made by people who observe you while you are working with someone else. Your manner, your sincere interest in the person you are training, your sense of humor, and your knowledge of your profession can all be seen plainly by anyone standing nearby.

Just as important is verbal communication. Trainers need to speak clearly, with a pleasant tone—preferably in clear and grammatically correct sentences! But being able to explain things logically is even more important. Trainers who consistently use correct terminology can help clients recognize and understand what they ought to be doing. Even so, problems can arise. Machine names may be incorrect or confusing. One company, for instance, labels a machine a "vertical pull" machine when it actually pulls horizontally. Most clients don't know much about weight machines, but they do know vertical from horizontal. The controversy concerning technical names as opposed to common names for muscles is often silly. Clients, unless they are heavy lifters, don't want to hear about or learn rectus abdominus, gastrocnemius, or biceps femoris when abs, calves, and hamstrings will do the job.

Listening

In order to be an effective communicator, you need to be a good listener. Effective listening is not the same as hearing. We are bombarded with noises throughout the day, but often do not consciously listen to all of the sounds around us. Listening is an active rather than a passive process. Half of all communication time is spent listening. Listening is

- receiving information through your ears (and eyes),
- giving meaning to that information,
- deciding what you think (or feel) about the information, and
- responding to what you hear (Bone, 1988).

You have to concentrate in order to listen effectively. How many times have you been involved in a conversation where the receiver was obviously not listening very well? It is frustrating, isn't it? No one likes to be avoided. Next time you are listening to someone, perhaps one of your clients, *pay attention* to what the other person is saying, *select* the part or parts of their message that is important for you, and *recognize* any emotional messages (e.g., embarrassment, soft or loud voice).

For an exercise on listening, try sitting quietly somewhere where people are around you, perhaps in the club, and listen to the voices and sounds around you. Write down what you remember. You may be surprised at how much you hear when you concentrate. One of the most important listening skills to learn is not to interrupt. Don't you hate it when someone constantly finishes your sentences for you? If you don't understand something, ask for clarification. Learning to be a good listener takes a conscious effort and practice. Are you a good listener? (See Table 10.2 and Figure 10.1.)

Assessing Your Clients

Part of effective communication is knowing as much as possible about the person you are communicating with. Clients come in all sizes, shapes, and attitudes. Some are whiners, some are lazy, some are skeptical. Some are hard workers and a joy to coach. Make it a point to study clients carefully, make an initial assessment, and try to remain open minded and flexible as you work. Find out their exercise background, both recent and over the past few years, and take a

Table 10.2 Characteristics of Poor and Good Listeners

Characteristics of a poor listener	Characteristics of a good listener
Always interrupts	Looks at the speaker
Jumps to conclusions	Asks questions to clarify
Finishes other people's sentences	Asks questions to show concern
Is inattentive, has wandering eyes, and uses poor posture	Repeats for clarity
Changes the subject	Does not rush
Writes everything down	Shows poise and emotional control
Doesn't give a response	Responds with a nod, smile, or frown
Is impatient	Pays close attention
Loses temper	Does not interrupt
Fidgets with pens, pencils, or paper clips	Keeps on the subject

Adapted from Montgomery (1981).

How Good a Listener Are You?

Instructions: Respond to each question according to the following scale:

1 = always
2 = frequently
3 = sometimes
4 = seldom
5 = never

_____ 1. I think about my own performance during an interaction, which results in my missing some of what the speaker has said.

_____ 2. I allow my mind to wander away from what the speaker is talking about.

_____ 3. I try to simplify messages I hear by omitting details.

_____ 4. I focus on a particular detail of what the speaker is saying instead of the general meanings the speaker wishes to communicate.

_____ 5. I allow my attitudes toward the topic or speaker to influence my evaluation of the message.

_____ 6. I hear what I expect to hear instead of what is actually being said.

_____ 7. I listen passively, letting the speaker do the work while I relax.

_____ 8. I listen to what others say, but I don't feel what they are feeling.

_____ 9. I evaluate what the speaker is saying before I fully understand the meanings intended.

_____ 10. I listen to the literal meanings that a speaker communicates, but do not look for hidden or underlying meanings.

Scoring

All the statements describe ineffective listening tendencies. High scores, therefore, reflect effective listening, and low scores reflect ineffective listening. If you scored significantly higher than 30, then you probably have better-than-average listening skills. Scores significantly below 30 represent lower-than-average listening skills.

Figure 10.1   Listening-skills test.
Reprinted from DeVito (1992).

medical history before you begin designing a program.

Talk to your clients; make it easy for them to open up. Many clients forget old injuries. Many will tell you they have never had any joint problems unless you ask specifically, "Have you ever had a knee problem?" Find out if they have ever done any vigorous exercise, if they have ever had physical therapy for an injury. Without prying, show some interest in their lives—their jobs, their families, their hobbies. Ask how they feel about exercise—whether they enjoy it, or consider it a chore, like taking medicine.

Most people like to talk about themselves, particularly when someone seems genuinely interested. When a 27-year-old man begins to tell you about some inconsequential bruise he got when he was 15, which meant he could not practice junior basketball and thus could not make the team, you may find out useful things about what motivates him. You will need to analyze, and perhaps discard a great deal of what you hear, but you have started to communicate.

After you determine a client's goals, be realistic about how long it will take to meet them and how much commitment will be required. When a 145-pound, 6'4" man tells you he wants to look like Arnold Schwarzenegger in 3 months, consider yourself obliged to tell him it's not going to happen. Be fair to him, and be fair to yourself! Give your clients a general overview of the program you propose for them. Tell them how much time is going to be necessary for optimum development in weight training, cardiovascular development, and desired weight gain or loss.

Be as specific as possible about the rate of progress the client can expect, taking into account problems such as injury, illness, job, or family commitments. A few trainers like to keep clients in the dark about what they are doing and why, in order to make the client dependent on them. (I find that reprehensible.) Clients will stay with you longer if you are open and honest about the progress they can expect.

Setting Goals

A goal is an end toward which you direct some specific effort. Essential elements of goals include

- an accomplishment to be achieved,
- a measurable outcome,
- a specific date and time to accomplish the goals, and
- a maximum cost (money or resources) allowed to achieve the goal.

Thus, a goal is a specific and measurable accomplishment to be achieved within specific time and cost constraints. Helping clients set realistic goals is one of the most important responsibilities of personal trainers.

Exercise programs should take the limits of the individual client into account. If the client is in very poor cardiovascular shape or has little muscular strength, you will obviously begin with a very easy program that aims at gradual improvement. One of the most important functions of the personal trainer is to help the client set short- and long-term goals that incorporate the *client's* objectives. Only after gathering and analyzing a lot of information about the client can you design a program to fit each client's objectives. Use Figure 10.2 to help you set goals.

Consider the steps outlined in the following case study as an example of goal setting.

Interview the Client

The client, Bob, is a 40-year-old executive who is in relatively good health, but he smokes and is 20-pounds overweight. Bob has come to Marcus, a personal trainer, because he wants to make some important lifestyle changes. Before helping Bob set some short-range and long-range goals, Marcus needs to assess Bob's current fitness level and his commitment to becoming more fit. Marcus and Bob discuss Bob's answers to the following questions:

1. What kinds of exercise programs have you tried in the past?
2. How much time do you have to commit to exercise?
3. What did you like most and least about your previous exercise programs?
4. What is your favorite exercise?
5. If you were to choose just one form of exercise, what would it be? Why?

After a careful discussion, Marcus determines that Bob has never stuck with an exercise program for very long. In the past, he has enjoyed skiing, playing tennis, walking, and riding his mountain bike. He feels he can realistically commit to 1 hour of exercise per day. Bob identifies his major fitness goals as quitting smoking and losing weight.

Develop Initial Program

Bob sets a date to quit smoking. He also agrees to attend a behavioral counseling program for people who have decided to quit smoking. His exercise program will start the same day as his smoking quit date, but Marcus and Bob both feel that Bob should wait to start his diet until he has 1 month of successful exercise training. Bob will attend 5 1-hour dietary counseling sessions with a registered dietitian, who will recommend a diet for him. His exercise program includes 4 days of aerobic exercise and 3 days of light weight training (see Figure 10.3). Marcus will see Bob 2 days a week and phone him 2 times per week.

Determine Short-Range Goals

Marcus and Bob write down these short-range goals for Bob:

1. Quit smoking on January 1.
2. Start attending smoking-cessation counseling on January 15.
3. Start an exercise program on January 1.
4. Start a diet on February 1.
5. Consult with a dietitian on January 23.
6. Reduce daily caloric intake.

Bob will have a caloric reduction of approximately 2 lbs per week, which is the recommended weight-loss range. It will take approximately 3 to 4 months for Bob to reach his goal weight if he sticks with his diet and exercise program.

---

1. What do you want to accomplish by entering a training program?

I want to lose 10 pounds.

---

2. Put this goal into a measurable form:

By August 26, 1995, I will lose 10 pounds by following the plan developed by my personal trainer.

---

3. Identify what you need to do to attain this goal:

In order to lose 10 pounds, I will follow the diet and exercise program outlined by my personal

trainer. I will commit to exercising at least 30-45 minutes 4-5 days per week.

4. List the activities necessary to carry out this plan of action:

Walk 30-45 minutes 4-5 days per week. Give up 3-4 of my favorite high-fat foods.

---

5. Review progress:

Every 2 weeks we will sit down and review my progress, making any changes necessary.

Figure 10.2   Sample goal-setting worksheet.

Determine Long-Range Goals

Some of Bob's most important long-range goals are to maintain his weight loss and his smoking cessation. Specific plans for Bob's long-range goals will be set after he achieves his short-range goals.

Reassessment

How often goals need to be reassessed depends on how often a client and trainer get together. In Bob's case, because quitting smoking and dieting are so difficult and are associated with a high degree of failure, Marcus will follow up with Bob frequently.

Motivation contracts (see Figure 10.4) are a fun and effective way to help clients stay focused on their goals. The contract clearly states the responsibilities of each party and can include some type of reward for reaching the client's goal. The contract should be reviewed on a regular basis to make necessary changes.

Motivating Clients

Unlike the skills you can teach clients, motivation cannot be taught. But it can be encouraged. Your job as a trainer is to design and conduct programs that help clients see what is possible, form some expectations about how much they can do, and then measure their progress. Small successes, and your praise for those successes, go a long way to motivate.

In golf, for example, the goal is to put the ball in the cup, using the smallest number of strokes. Small successes along the way, such as par on the ninth hole, are often enough to fan the embers of motivation, which keeps the golfer going even when the overall score is nowhere close to par. In the same way, the loss of 1 inch from a 40-inch waistline or 5 pounds from a 200-pound body have kept many a faltering exerciser coming back to the gym for more, because the client can measure and see the results. A 1/4-inch increase in the size of a biceps can send a beginning weightlifter into spasms of ecstasy. Help clients keep track of their weight and measurements—waist, chest, hips, and thighs—and you help them stay on track and achieve their goals. To these measurements I add blood pressure and resting pulse rate. I take measurements early in a client's training program and keep them up to date.

Some skills are easily measured, such as time for a 50-yard dash. Others, the strength of a wrist and

Cardiovascular Workout

Week	Warm-up (min)	Time (min)	Pace (mph)	Heart rate (% of max)	Cool-down (min)
1	5-7	20	2.5	60	5-7
2	5-7	30	3.0	65	5-7
3	5-7	40	3.0	70	5-7
4	5-7	50	3.5	75	5-7

Strength-Training Workout

Exercise	Reps	Sets
Leg extensions	10-12	1
Hip extension	10-12	1
Leg curl	10-12	1
Push-ups	10-15	1
Bench press	10-15	1
Biceps curls	10-12	1
Modified squats	10-15	1
Modified curl-ups	10-15	3

Figure 10.3 Sample exercise program.

hand-eye coordination, for instance, are difficult or impossible to measure quantitatively. Pictures of body types or of performers in related fields or skills and reading materials about the benefits of staying fit can all be good motivating tools.

During my first 6 months in California, I worked with an exotic dancer. She began by bringing in photographs of Madonna and Linda Hamilton and saying, "That's how I want to look." Some of the muscles in question were easily measurable, while others were not, but periodically we pulled out the pictures from her exercise folder and visually assessed her progress. (So did the other members of the club.) The moral? Use whatever works. And of course, there is the positive reinforcement you provide. Recently, I worked with a group of three businessmen. After the third workout, I noticed they were all working a little more diligently and wondered if their efforts were the result of getting to know each other and me better. I spoke to each of them privately, and all three said that my positive comments made the difference and that their previous trainer had never complimented them.

While it is easy to measure weight loss on a scale, a change in the ratio of fat to lean is much harder to measure. Decreasing body measurements have calmed many irate clients who realize that not only have they not lost weight, but that they have gained a few pounds. If their measurements show a smaller waist, hips, or thighs, they realize they have actually lost fat, gained muscle, and altered their body builds.

Most health clubs do not have human performance laboratories with sophisticated equipment and testers, and cardiovascular assessment ranges from poor to nonexistent. Even under ideal conditions, cardiovascular assessments can be influenced by factors such as lack of sleep, illness, stress, and eating too close to testing time. In addition, the skills of the tester, the apparatus used, and whether the activity has to be interrupted to do the test also affect the accuracy of measurements. I most often use a treadmill and heart monitor, because with a heart monitor the client doesn't have to stop the activity for me to take a reading. This is another

This contract is made this day, _____, 19__ between Bob Smith and Marcus Jones.

I, Bob Smith, agree to:

1. Quit smoking on January 1.
2. Attend at least 90% of my smoking-cessation counseling appointments.
3. Start and stick with an exercise program that consists of at least 4 days of walking or riding my mountain bike for up to 1 hour per session, and 20 to 30 minutes of weight training 3 days per week.
4. Stay on a 750-kcal-per-day reduction diet until I have lost 20 pounds.
5. Agree to weigh myself only 1 time per week.
6. Meet with a dietitian on 5 separate occasions.
7. Exercise with my personal trainer in person 2 times per week and talk to him on the phone 2 times per week.
8. Call my personal trainer if I am having trouble or if I have questions regarding my exercise program.
9. Call my personal trainer if I need to miss a training session.
10. Carefully follow the instructions given to me by my personal trainer.

If I achieve my weight-loss goals and remain smoke free for 6 months, I am going to treat myself to:

_____

I, Marcus Jones, agree to:

1. Clearly explain the rationale for the program established for my client.
2. Show my client how to exercise safely.
3. Design a safe and effective program for my client.
4. Be available to answer questions and offer emotional support for my client.
5. Be a good listener.

This contract will be evaluated on _____, 19__.

Signed:

_____   _____
Client   Date

_____   _____
Personal trainer   Date

_____   _____
Witness   Date

Figure 10.4 Sample motivational contract.

reason I believe heart rate monitors should be standard equipment for personal trainers—particularly when you are training pregnant women, overweight clients, people recovering from illness or surgery, or (at the other end of the fitness spectrum) high-level athletes.

Clients can be motivated by things as trivial as a gold star, a small trophy, recognition from other club members, pictures on club bulletin boards, or their trainers' words of praise. The methods of motivation are limited only by the trainer's ingenuity.

Summary

Successful personal trainers are effective teachers, communicators, listeners, and motivators. Too often personal trainers concentrate on signing new clients, keeping abreast of news in the field, and making sure clients achieve their goals; they often overlook the personal side of personal training. Personal training is a *people* business, which requires good *people* skills. Personal trainers need to take time to consistently improve their teaching and communication skills; the rewards will soon become evident.

Bibliography

Bone, D. (1988). *The business of listening.* Los Altos, CA: Crisp Publications.

Burgoon, M., & Ruffner, M. (1974). *Human communication.* New York: Holt, Rinehart & Winston.

Decker, B. (1988). *The art of communication.* Los Altos, CA: Crisp.

DeVito, J.A. (1992). *The interpersonal communication book.* New York: HarperCollins.

Montgomery, R. (1981). *Listening made easy.* New York: AMACOM.

Chapter 11

Designing Individualized Exercise Programs

Douglas Brooks

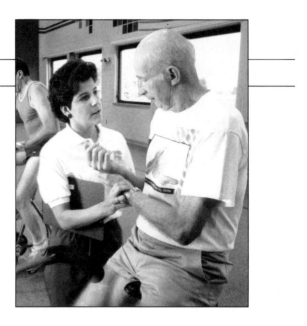

The objectives of this chapter are to

- discuss important aspects of designing exercise programs,
- explain how to conduct an effective interview,
- suggest ways to start a client on a safe program, and
- discuss prescreening tests and objectives.

Overview

Designing exercise programs for individuals is both an art and a science. The scientific part is usually the easier part; the art of program design is the challenge. How do you design the most effective and appropriate exercise program for someone? One way is by first listening to the needs of the individual. The initial client interview will help you plan a safe and effective exercise program, based on the needs of individual clients. With time, trainers learn to develop more creative exercise programs. This chapter presents essential information on the art and science of program design. It reviews important procedures to follow before starting someone on an exercise program and concludes with some great ways to make exercise programs more creative and effective.

Program design may well be your biggest challenge as a personal trainer. Even when you are designing exercise programs for healthy, asymptomatic people, there are many considerations. It doesn't take long to realize that one-size-fits-all program design does not work. Every individual has unique needs, interests, and responses to various activities. Whether or not you are an experienced personal trainer, you probably have questions about program design. Although theory is a prerequisite to creative and effective exercise programming, even personal trainers armed with theoretical information may wonder what the practical solutions are to their clients' individual programming needs.

After training an average of 40 to 50 clients a week for the past 9 years, I've learned to blend the usable and practical aspects of theory into the reality of day-to-day personal training. You can simplify your own program design procedures, and ensure consistent quality, by using the following plan.

Preexercise Health Screening

With proper information gathering, you will know your clients' current health status and their interests and fitness needs. The information-gathering process should include a medical history/health questionnaire, a client interview, and fitness testing (optional).

The Medical History/Health Questionnaire

The medical history/health questionnaire (see Figure 11.1) (ACSM, 1991; ACE, 1991; Brooks, 1990; Francis & Francis, 1988; Golding, 1989; and Heyward, 1991 all contain examples) should ask questions regarding

- medical concerns, such as blood pressure, smoking, blood-lipid profile, orthopaedic and cardiovascular history, allergies, medications, last physical examinations, and family histories;
- the client's personal understanding of basic fitness concepts, such as cardiovascular fitness and safe weight loss;
- current and past fitness activities;
- goals and interests;
- dietary information, such as eating habits; and
- lifestyle and stress profile, indicating such aspects as job type and personality traits.

Your questionnaire should ask only for information that you understand and can use to determine your client's course of action.

The purpose of a health evaluation is to detect the presence of disease. According to Heyward (1991), a comprehensive health evaluation should include a medical history questionnaire, coronary risk factor analysis, a physical examination, laboratory tests, and medical clearance. Based on the results, individuals are classified as apparently healthy, at risk, or with disease.

According to the American College of Sports Medicine (1991), prospective participants should obtain a physical examination and medical clearance from a physician, especially if they are men over 40 years or women over 50 years of age; at higher risk (individuals who have one or more coronary risk factors or symptoms of cardiopulmonary or metabolic disease); or known to have cardiovascular, pulmonary, or metabolic disorders. ACSM recommends a maximal exercise test for healthy older men (> 40 yrs) and women (> 50 yrs) before beginning a vigorous (> 60% functional aerobic capacity) exercise program. These tests should be administered with physician supervision and conducted by exercise technicians who are well-trained and experienced in monitoring exercise tests and emergencies. Moderate exercise (exercise intensity 40-60% $\dot{V}O_2$ max) without maximal stress testing may be appropriate for older clients. Moderate exercise is an exercise intensity well within the individual's current capacity. It can be comfortably sustained for a prolonged period of time and is generally noncompetitive.

When something on the health history questionnaire appears to be out of the ordinary, I consider it a red flag that needs some kind of attention or follow-up beyond my expertise. A few examples of red flags are age of the individual (i.e., over 40 years of age for men and over 50 years of age for women), history of heart disease, orthopaedic concerns, high blood pressure, pregnancy, and diabetes. It could also signify an area where you simply need more information before you can begin to create the best and safest program possible for your client.

If you have any questions or hesitations concerning the safety of proceeding with an individual's program, check with your client's physician or health care provider. You begin to see the importance of the information-gathering phase and establishing a relationship with your client's health care provider. Proper written and verbal (interview) screening of your client reduces the risk of assuming liability and putting your client in dangerous situations. Ask the right questions!

Name _____

Address _____

Home Phone _____ Business Phone _____

Age _____ Birthdate _____ Social Security # _____

Physician's Name _____ Phone _____

Health History

1. Do you smoke? _____ How much? _____

2. Has your doctor ever said your blood pressure was too high or low? _____

3. Do you have any known cardiovascular problems (abnormal ECG, previous heart attack, atherosclerosis, etc.)? _____ If so, what? _____

4. Has your doctor ever told you your cholesterol level was high? _____

5. Are you overweight? _____ How much? _____

6. Do you have any injuries or orthopaedic problems (bursitis, bad back, bad knees, etc.)? _____

   _____

7. Are you taking any prescribed medications or dietary supplements? _____

   _____

8. Date of last physical examination _____

9. Do you have any other medical conditions or problems not previously mentioned? _____

   _____

10. Are you currently involved in a regular exercise program? _____

    If yes, please describe _____

11. What are your goals within this program? _____

    _____

Consent Form

I acknowledge, to the best of my ability, that I am in good health and have no known medical problems that would restrict my ability to participate in this exercise program.

Signed _____ Date _____

Figure 11.1 Sample screening form.
Reprinted from Brooks (1990).

The Client Interview

The initial client interview is the beginning of a continuing dialogue. It initially allows you to gather facts regarding your client's interests, needs, wants, and understanding of fitness from a health standpoint. This type of interaction continues throughout most successful personal trainer–client relationships, and allows you to find out what the client wants to accomplish. It is important to acknowledge the clients' perspectives on how to achieve fitness and give them ownership and responsibility for their fitness programs. It sends a very important signal that you are listening as well. This intrinsic motivation will go a long way in exciting your client to be compliant because you have invited the client to be involved.

In creating a balanced program for your clients, it is easy to incorporate their interests into a program that covers their health and fitness needs. Your clients must always remain a part of the process. Their input and feelings are the most important components in directing your program design.

Fitness Testing

Fitness testing (ACE, 1991; ACSM, 1991; Brooks, 1990; Fair, 1992; Golding, 1989; Heyward, 1991; Jackson & Pollock, 1985; Kendall, McCreary, & Provance, 1993; McArdle, Katch, & Katch, 1991; Sharkey, 1990) is an optional motivational tool that many trainers use to excite their clients about improvement in their fitness over time. Fitness testing is not a diagnostic tool that assesses the diseased or nondiseased status of an individual. Nor is it a tool to determine your client's readiness to engage in activity. A properly designed health questionnaire, along with a relationship with your client's health care professional, is the way to determine your client's readiness level.

Personal trainers typically test submaximal cardiorespiratory fitness, muscle strength and endurance, and flexibility. All the current models for testing have both strengths and weaknesses in their abilities to assess improvements in the different areas of fitness. Personal trainers should mostly be concerned with whether the tests are appropriate to the individual client (in terms of safety and fitness needs) and whether they reflect balanced fitness. The second criterion applies especially to tests for muscle strength and endurance, and flexibility. As part of the screening process, I encourage personal trainers to administer skinfold (Brooks, 1990; Golding, 1989; Heyward, 1991; Jackson & Pollock, 1985; McArdle, Katch, & Katch, 1991; Lohman, Roche, & Martorell, 1988) and at least resting blood pressure measurements (Brooks; Golding; Heyward). Both are simple skills to learn and safe to administer.

Skinfold Measurements.   Skinfold measurement is an effective motivator to demonstrate safe fat loss and effective exercise design. The measurements may be used to predict a percentage of body fat. They can also be used to predict improvements in body composition for the individual client, based solely on changes in the skinfold measurements themselves (see Figure 11.2). I prefer using the process shown in Figure 11.2 because all of the changes are specifically relevant to the individual client. In predicting a percentage of body fat, your clients are likely to compare themselves with others. For people who are lean and fit this can be an exciting motivator;

however, for overfat individuals, this comparison can be a powerful form of negative feedback.

Blood Pressure.   High blood pressure or hypertension is often a symptomless disease that influences the progression of various vascular diseases, including coronary heart disease. Early detection of hypertension and consistent monitoring of blood pressure may help your client avoid symptomatic vascular disease (i.e., heart attack, stroke, claudication) in later life. In concert with your client's physician, helping a client monitor blood pressure can be an invaluable service.

Flexibility and Postural Assessment.   Trainers must begin to go beyond the simple sit-and-reach test to assess flexibility. Some experts (Kendall, McCreary, & Provance, 1993; Plowman, 1992) are beginning to question whether the test can be administered safely to a variety of populations and whether it gives any specific or valuable information about flexibility in the low back and hamstrings muscle groups.

Flexibility is joint specific, which implies that a battery of flexibility tests are needed to adequately evaluate your client's range of motion needs. Postural assessment or analysis is essential to inform clients whether their alignment is normal or whether they have postural imperfections. Poor posture can place an excessive burden on bones, joints, muscles, tendons, and ligaments. Therefore, it is important to identify any significant postural imperfections that might predispose your client to injuries. Improvements in posture can involve several different parts of the body. Correcting only a single misalignment will be unsuccessful. Effective programming must include a number of stretching and strengthening exercises for the affected body parts (Brooks, 1990; Francis & Francis, 1988; Kendall, McCreary, & Provance, 1993; Plowman, 1992).

Finally, a few words of caution for any of the assessment tests you choose to use. If the test has the potential to be an embarrassment to the client, don't use it. For example, if you are working with an extremely overfat individual, is it really necessary to administer any tests to establish that the person is overfat, has a low cardiorespiratory status, and has flexibility and postural imbalances? A visual check and conversation will detail all of this. Administer tests only when they have the potential for positive feedback. It isn't very motivating for an obese individual to be told the the jaws of the skinfold caliper won't open wide enough to allow a measurement. Stay sensitive to your clients!

A fitness test should not be used if it puts your client in an inappropriate, dangerous, or high-risk

1. **Sum = relative degree of fatness (individual)***
2. **Body fat distribution specific to site measurement****
3. **Before and after percent change of sum and individual measures*****

Fatfolds (mm)	Before	After	Change	% Change***
Triceps**	22.5	19.4	−3.1	−13.8
Subscapular**	19.0	17.0	−2.0	−10.5
Suprailiac**	34.5	30.2	−4.3	−12.5
Abdomen**	33.7	29.4	−4.3	−12.8
Thigh**	21.6	18.7	−2.9	−13.4
Sum*	131.3*	114.7	−16.6	−12.6

Note. ***Percent change = Change divided by Before
Example: −13.8 = −3.1 divided by 22.5 × (100)

Figure 11.2 How to use skinfold scores without predicting percent body fat.

situation, as related to their current fitness and health status. For example, can you see the absurdity of maximally testing an individual who is just beginning a strength program to determine their starting weights? This scenario depicts a situation where the trainer may have elected to follow a standard recipe regardless of the client's current physical and mental needs. It is easy to fall into ruts based on nothing more than tradition or convenience. It should be reemphasized that fitness testing is never an absolute necessity. The keys to a safe and effective start-up program are administering a proper health questionnaire and establishing a liaison with your client's physician or attending health care professional. However, you are encouraged to learn these assessment skills, which will become additional tools in your total fitness package.

Initial and Follow-Up Fitness Assessments. Timing for initial fitness assessments depends primarily on the needs of the client. Remember, fitness assessments are not diagnostic in nature. Thus, unlike a physician's evaluation, fitness assessments do not give you any information that is crucial to beginning a safe program. For many of your clients, it is prudent to create a foundation of conditioning before testing, especially if you choose to assess your clients with tests that require activity.

Retesting coincides nicely with the phases of initial conditioning, improvement, and maintenance as described by the American College of Sports Medicine (1991). The greatest gains in conditioning in a properly designed program will be in the first 4 to 6 weeks. Maintenance conditioning can begin around 6 months. Retesting 6 to 8 weeks after the initial test makes sense from a physiological and adaptation standpoint. You also stand to motivate your clients when they can measure improvements. Testing again at 6 months, 1 year, and thereafter yearly is a reasonable plan to follow.

Prepare your clients for success by explaining the phases of initial conditioning, improvement, and maintenance. Remember that maintenance is not regression, but is a positive position reflecting your client's happiness with the current program and health and fitness level. When maintenance is presented in a positive manner, this creates a realistic view of the improvements your client can expect to make over a period of time. Discussing the philosophy of maintenance cuts short the potential for failed expectations and the unrealistic notion that one's gains in fitness will continue to be as dramatic as in their first 4 to 6 weeks of training. It reflects your professionalism and knowledge by anticipating the normal occurrence of plateaued fitness gains.

Physical Programming

Once you have a thorough understanding and current physical history of your client, the next step is physical programming. Physical programming involves three key areas:

1. Cardiorespiratory conditioning
2. Muscle strength and muscle endurance conditioning
3. Flexibility training and postural awareness

When creating programs, you should differentiate between training for athletic performance and creating fitness and health improvements. Your approach and time investment will be different in each area.

You must approach your client's needs and goals with a specific, well-planned, accurate program. You must know what overloads change the body's energy and its musculoskeletal systems. Overload refers to the frequency, intensity, and duration levels during a workout. To improve health and fitness, the overload must require more effort than the body is accustomed to. This knowledge enables you to manipulate the many variables that affect positive adaptations in the cardiorespiratory, muscle strength and endurance, and flexibility components of fitness.

Cardiorespiratory Conditioning

Cardiorespiratory conditioning enhances the delivery of blood (heart and blood vessels) and the extraction of oxygen (skeletal muscle capillaries). More important, it ensures an adequate supply and use of oxygen for most of the body's functions.

The overload definition and type of activity necessary for change is a rhythmic, continuous, large-muscle activity that promotes a simultaneous increase in heart rate and return of blood (venous return) to the heart. Frequency, intensity and duration are important considerations. It is generally recommended that clients exercise 3 to 5 times per week, at 40% to 85% of their $\dot{V}O_2$ max (which compares to 55-90% of maximum heart rate) for 20 to 60 minutes (ACSM, 1991). However, considerably less exercise has significant impact on decreasing morbidity (disease and illness) and mortality (death) (ACSM, 1991; Blair, Kohl, Paffenbarger, Clark, Cooper, & Gibbons, 1989). Moderate exercise can affect the health of an individual significantly. Training for high levels of fitness and performance is very different than engaging in activity to enhance health and well-being. In designing programs for healthy, average populations, many trainers err on the side of creating workouts that are too hard. Listen to your client's goals and carefully look at their current fitness levels.

Perceived exertion is a good way to determine how hard a client should work. For general health gains, a person should be comfortably uncomfortable. Use the talk test. The client should be able to utter three to five words without gasping when performing rhythmic, continuous activity.

Muscle Strength and Endurance Conditioning

The general guideline for change (proper overload) is a progressive increase in resistance over time, challenging all the movements that the muscles make. A progressive increase in resistance is necessary for continued increases in muscle strength and endurance, and for gradual increases in intensity. All the movements of the body must be challenged to ensure balanced strength between opposing muscle groups.

A safe starting resistance for most clients is one that allows completion of at least 12 to 20 repetitions. This intensity equates to less than 70% of one repetition maximum (1 RM) and is generally a safe starting intensity for most people. I prefer not to initially test a client's ability to lift his or her maximum weight one time (1 RM) and then calculate a percentage of this maximum lift to determine starting weight. The contradiction is obvious. The unprepared client is put in a high-risk, maximal performance situation. This situation totally ignores the progressive adaptation principle. I would prefer to err on the side of using too little, rather than too much, weight to determine starting points.

By referring to Table 11.1, you can observe that a resistance or load that causes the body's musculature to fatigue between 8 to 12 repetitions is a moderate load. This equates to 70% to 80% of any individual's 1 RM. For a more fit person or a client whose goal is to maximize muscle size and strength gain, this is an appropriate load to progress to. Notice that I have not mentioned how much weight should be lifted. Research indicates that a 1 RM lift equates to about 75% of a person's maximum lifting capacity for any given lift. This intensity seems necessary to optimize muscular strength and hypertrophy gains. The starting load is determined by an appropriate resistance that fatigues the muscle within the stated repetition goal range. The *goal range* is determined by a variety of factors that include the person's current fitness level specific to resistance training, exercise history, and stated resistance-training goals (i.e., muscle endurance or muscle hypertrophy).

Resistance-Training Systems. There is also a myriad of resistance-training systems. A system in resistance training is defined as any combination of sets, repetitions, and loads (weight or resistance). Systems are often designed to address specific and sometimes nonspecific training goals. Therefore, specific combinations of sets, repetitions, and loads often promise exciting results. This leads to the often asked question: What system—how many repetitions and sets, or how much resistance—is best?

Table 11.1 Specificity Chart

Relative loading	Outcome	%1 RM	Range of repetitions	Number of sets	Rest between sets
Light	Muscular endurance	<70	12-20	2-3	20-30 s
Moderate	Hypertrophy	70-80	8-12	3-6	30-90 s
Heavy	Maximum strength	80-100	1-8	3-5+	2-5 min

Adapted from Baechle and Groves (1992).

Most systems, regardless of their format, are effective. Any stimulus that is introduced to a client who isn't accustomed to it will cause the client's body to adapt to the new overload. This produces a training effect. Fortunately, in spite of how we train ourselves or others, we sometimes still get results. Whether the method meets your client's needs and safety concerns is another story. Table 11.1 summarizes the types of results you can expect for various relative loads (intensities).

Intensity. To optimize strength increases, resistance-training workouts should strive to recruit fast-twitch (FT) motor units because their biochemical and physical characteristics are suited to enhance muscle hypertrophy and nervous system adaptations that enhance strength gains. Initially this means that someone just starting a program is encouraged to fatigue the muscle in about 12 to 20 repetitions. The experienced or more fit person might strive for muscle failure between 8 to 12 repetitions. This intensity of exercise is likely to optimize FT motor unit recruitment and optimize strength adaptations.

High-repetition sets (i.e., greater than 20 repetitions) do not generally provide sufficient stimulus to make the muscle grow significantly in size, to improve the efficiency of the nervous system (motor learning), or to increase strength. Low-intensity (high-repetition) exercise will not greatly stimulate FT muscle fibers, and stimulating the metabolic characteristics of these fibers is conducive to gains in muscle strength and size.

Just how much control do we really have in directing muscular strength and endurance results? Genetics, as related to muscle fiber type, number of fibers, and neural and hormonal influences, ultimately determines the outer ranges of strength and body shape. However, each person's optimal potential, as defined by genetics, can best be reached when the trainer

- designs resistance-training systems with specific goals in mind;

- fits all systems into the specificity chart (see Table 11.1);
- encourages consistent, regular, and varied efforts;
- teaches correct exercise technique (biomechanics);
- allows for the recovery/building process; and
- keeps accurate records.

No program or exercise guideline is written in stone. Err on the side of conservatism. You must know your client's physical limits and perception of what is too much. Intensity is relative to the individual. Don't join the ranks of many trainers who create programs that are too hard for their clients. Even if you don't injure them, you surely will defeat them.

Flexibility

Flexibility may be defined as the range of motion about a joint. It is specific to each joint. Being flexible in one joint does not influence flexibility in another joint. The guideline for change is a static (no bouncing), sustained (10 to 60 seconds) stretch, held to the point of mild tension. The recommended frequency is 3 to 7 times per week. There are different types of stretching and varying combinations of these. However, when the risk versus effectiveness ratio is examined between each, the static, sustained stretch gives you the most for your efforts. If your client's goal is to attain functional flexibility, this goal can easily and effectively be achieved with static stretching.

Static, active, passive, and proprioceptive neuromuscular facilitation (PNF), or facilitated stretching, all yield favorable results. I recommend using PNF techniques with participants who are fairly fit and aware of their bodies. However, PNF stretches are commonly used with a variety of clients, ranging from the deconditioned to the athlete. Safely teaching PNF stretches requires you to have a clear understanding of neurophysiology, a real sense of the limits of a client's body, and constant verbal and nonverbal communication with the client. Be sure you are properly trained and have adequate knowledge before introducing this technique. Remember, clients can achieve very acceptable flexibility gains with static stretches, which are less likely to cause injuries.

Active Rest Concept

Regardless of fitness level, I generally weave the concept of active rest throughout my fitness routines. The active rest concept uses sequences of chosen exercises to structure a workout that optimizes time availability and accommodates the fitness level of the individual. Typically, a large amount of time in traditional fitness programs involves recovery from work performed. There are several ways to minimize wasted recovery time, or to eliminate it.

1. Use perceived exertion and intervals (work, recovery) to keep your client in motion during cardiorespiratory conditioning.
2. Sequence resistance-training exercises so that they alternate from muscle group to muscle group or from upper to lower body to the trunk.
3. If a muscle group is targeted for consecutive multiple sets, the recovery phases(s) can be used for flexibility training.

For the trainer looking for maximum results, this combination is a great way to optimize your limited time with the typical client. Your programs should differentiate between training for athletic performance and creating functional health improvements, because each demands its own approaches and time investments. Where does your client fit?

Cross-Training

Now that your base approach is set, the fun continues. By first understanding overload and how different overloads specifically cause changes in the body's systems, the world of programming choices becomes less confusing. Simply apply the definitions of overload for each component of fitness to any type of training, and this will reveal the component(s) of fitness you are training. A person may cross-train within a component of fitness, such as cardiorespiratory fitness (running, walking, stepping), or between components of fitness (e.g., circuit training with muscular endurance and cardiorespiratory fitness emphasized). Utilizing cross-training within your program gives you five big advantages:

1. Variety and change
2. New physiological stimulation resulting in new fitness gains
3. Motivation
4. Compliance ("sticking with it")
5. Decreasing likelihood of overuse and overtraining injuries occurring from repeated, repetitive stresses

Some clients like change and some don't. Exercise variety is important for all of the previously mentioned reasons. However, the timing of its implementation is directly related to the client's need, and more importantly, readiness for change. Too often, we as trainers initiate the change because we need a change. Instead, it is wisest to first consider the client's physical needs, but it is even more important to judge a client's desire and mental readiness for change.

Individual Needs for Healthy Clients

All of your clients have special concerns. As you continue to fulfill their needs, your perceived value as a trainer increases. You have already solved the problem of balanced fitness by working on cardiorespiratory fitness, muscular strength and endurance, and flexibility fitness. You will need to consider issues such as performance versus fitness versus health, safe weight control, strength plateaus, and perinatal concerns.

You will also need to address new training ideas, such as lateral training, plyometrics, step training, step circuits, and fitness walking. To evaluate these methods, apply the overload definitions for each component of fitness. Start by asking a question such as, Does this activity supply rhythmic, sustained, large-muscle–group activity that simultaneously supports an increased heart rate and return of blood to the heart? This process clarifies what system(s) is being challenged by each activity in question.

Success

Ensuring the client's perception of success is one, if not the most, important aspect of program design. Four factors ensure exercise adherence (and a successful business for you).

1. Time—keep beginning workouts under 1 hour, 2 to 3 times a week.
2. Variety—use cross-training when appropriate.

3. Intrinsic motivation—both you and your clients should know why they want to exercise (ask them!).
4. Lifestyle changes—people must like what they are doing to incorporate the new behavior into their daily routines.

Success in terms of proper program design means a healthy, happy client, as well as a thriving business. Most people do not want to exercise hard. Most exercise to feel better and have more energy for daily living. We as trainers need to step out of our own heads and walk into the heads of our clients. Most of our clients would not plan their exercise programs like you plan your own. Consider this thought seriously, and you are on your way to effective and safe program design!

The Reality Factor

I have worked with some of my personal training clients for as long as 9 years. Many still do not perform with perfect exercise technique. Some do not have all of the ideal components of a balanced fitness program comfortably integrated into their daily schedule. Others have never linked their moderate cardiorespiratory interval segments into a continuous effort. Most will never experience proprioceptive neuromuscular facilitation stretching in its true, intense form.

Though the majority of clients are not the perfect models of textbook programming, their individual improvement is great. Their lives are better. I practice personal training using techniques that are specific and individualized to my client's goals, physical abilities, and readiness to learn. I attempt to optimize my client's involvement in fitness for a lifetime, with whatever techniques it takes. That means not becoming a robotic trainer who uses one recipe or program for every client. Fitness programming at best is vague. More often than not, an effective program and successful business offers a smorgasbord of options that meet your clients' changing needs. Remember to emphasize the goal of progress, not perfection.

Going Beyond Physical Activity

Personal trainers must look beyond activity only to a broader health-issues perspective. Assessing and addressing coronary risk factors is a first step in increasing your perceived value to your client. Do you help your client implement behavior changes related to a stressful lifestyle, a family history of coronary heart disease, obesity, lack of regular exercise, smoking, high blood pressure, high cholesterol or high-density-lipoprotein–cholesterol ratio? If you can direct your client toward improvement in any of these potential problem areas, you have taken the step of going beyond being an "exercise mechanic." In other words, machinery and physical activity are not your only approaches to a healthy and balanced lifestyle.

Clients With Special Needs

Special-need populations and high-risk conditions that trainers might encounter include cardiac rehabilitation, obesity, neurological and chronic degenerative diseases, diabetes, asthma, youth, aging, and women requiring perinatal care. When you first encounter a special-needs client, you will have to answer the question, Do I have the abilities and desire to work with this person? The keys to working with a high-risk clientele are to work within the scope of your training and to receive guidance or an exercise prescription from a qualified professional, such as a physician, osteopathic doctor, physical therapist, chiropractor, or registered dietitian.

What is within the scope of your practice? If you completely understand the necessary precautions or modifications recommended by the client's health care provider and you feel you can adhere to them, then you are probably capable of working with that client. If you don't understand a training principle, are unfamiliar with the condition, or are not confident about the training regimen, then you should refer the client elsewhere.

Summary

Bringing your skills and training back to a personal level includes an ongoing dialogue with your clients and exhibiting people skills that communicate, "I care about you." This is best shown by your detailed attention to your clients' needs, your professional growth and behavior, and your delivery of impeccable service. You should have the ability to charm, cajole, educate, and prod when necessary. You should not only convince and assist clients in achieving their exercise goals, but also help them sustain their level of enthusiasm and commitment to health-related lifestyle changes and regular exercise.

References

American College of Sports Medicine. (1990). *Recommended quantity and quality of exercise for developing and maintaining cardiorespiratory and muscular fitness in healthy adults.* (Available from the American College of Sports Medicine).

American College of Sports Medicine. (1991). *Guidelines for exercise testing and prescription* (4th ed.). Philadelphia: Lea & Febiger.

American Council on Exercise. (1991). *Personal trainer manual.* San Diego: Author.

Baechle, T., & Groves, B. (1992). *Weight training—Steps to success.* Champaign, IL: Human Kinetics.

Blair, S., Kohl, H.W., Paffenbarger, R.S., Clark, D.G., Cooper, K.H., & Gibbons, L.W. (1989, November). Physical fitness and all-cause mortality: A prospective study of healthy men and women. *Journal of the American Medical Association,* **262,** 2395-2401.

Brooks, D. (1990). *Going solo—The art of personal training* (2nd ed.). Mammoth Lakes, CA: Moves International.

Fair, E. (1992, June). Fitness software. *IDEA Today,* p. 27.

Francis, P., & Francis, L. (1988). *If it hurts, don't do it.* Rocklin, CA: Prima Publishing.

Golding, L. (1989). *The Y's way to physical fitness.* Champaign, IL: Human Kinetics.

Heyward, V. (1991). *Advanced fitness assessment & exercise prescription* (2nd ed.). Champaign, IL: Human Kinetics.

Jackson, A.S., & Pollock, M. (1985). Practical assessment of body composition. *The Physician and Sportsmedicine,* **13**(5), 76-90.

Kendall, F., McCreary, E., & Provance, P. (1993). *Muscles—Testing and function* (4th ed.). Baltimore: Williams and Wilkins.

Lohman, T., Roche, A.F., & Martorell, R. (1988). *Anthropometric standardization reference manual.* Champaign, IL: Human Kinetics.

McArdle, W.D., Katch, F.I., & Katch, V.L. (1991). *Exercise physiology—Energy, nutrition, and human performance* (3rd ed.). Philadelphia: Lea & Febiger.

Plowman, S. (1992). Physical activity, physical fitness, and low back pain. *Exercise and Sport Sciences Reviews,* **20,** 221-242.

Sharkey, B. (1990). *Physiology of fitness* (3rd ed.). Champaign, IL: Human Kinetics.

Professional Organizations, Resources, and Certifications

Service Literature

Corporate Wellness: Its Bottom-Line Impact

Wellness Councils of America
7101 Newport Ave., Suite 311
Omaha, NE 68152

Annually updated results summarized from America's finest companies on the cost-benefits of corporate health promotion programs. Free.

Health Fitness Brochures

David N. Camaione, Ph.D.,
  FACSM
University of Connecticut
Center for Health Fitness
359 Mansfield Road
Storrs, CT 06269

A collection of concisely written brochures on health fitness topics, including 1) Exercise as a means of controlling stress. 2) Exercise, weight control and calories. 3) Exercise facts and fallacies. 4) The benefits of exercise. 5) Circuit training. 6) Coronary risk profile. 7) Exercise: How much is enough. 8) Health fitness assessment for public safety personnel. $7.50.

How to Begin Your Exercise Program

IDEA
6190 Cornerstone Court E.,
Suite 204
San Diego, CA 92121

A pamphlet describing a three-step plan to start exercising, tips for sticking to it, a planning worksheet and common exercise myths. Free.

How to Choose a Quality Aerobic Fitness Instructor

IDEA
6190 Cornerstone Court E.,
Suite 204
San Diego, CA 92121

A pamphlet detailing a checklist of questions to ask when evaluating instructors. Free.

How to Choose a Quality Fitness Facility

IDEA
6190 Cornerstone Court E.,
Suite 204
San Diego, CA 92121

A pamphlet detailing a checklist of questions to ask when evaluating fitness facilities. Free.

Note. Reprinted with permission of *Fitness Management.*

How To Choose a Quality Personal Trainer

IDEA
6190 Cornerstone Court E.,
Suite 204
San Diego, CA 92121

A pamphlet detailing a checklist of questions to ask when evaluating personal trainers. Free.

Soccer Sports Medicine

Dr. Donald T. Kirkendall
Illinois State University
Horton Fieldhouse, Room 214
Normal, IL 61761

Assistance in searching literature on soccer sports medicine topics, from the American Medical Soccer Association bibliographer. Free.

10 Exercises You Shouldn't Do

Pro-Fit
12012-156th Ave. S.E.
Renton, WA 98059

A list of exercises to avoid or modify. Also includes a list of 10 exercises most people need. Free.

Periodicals

American Fitness

American Fitness
15250 Ventura Blvd., Suite 200
Sherman Oaks, CA 91403

A bi-monthly magazine, published by the Aerobics and Fitness Associaiton of America, featuring health and fitness information for the consumer. $27/year.

American Journal of Health Promotion

American Journal of Health
    Promotion
746 Purdy St.
Birmingham, MI 48009

A quarterly journal of research, reviews, editorials and resources in worksite wellness and public health. $59.95/year.

AWHP's Worksite Health

Association for Worksite Health Promotion
60 Revere Drive, Suite 500
Northbrook, IL 60062

A quarterly magazine for members of AWHP. Case studies, indepth interviews and research studies are designed to educate and inform health professionals and decision-makers on the efficacy of worksite health programs. Price included in membership.

CBI

IRSA
The Association of Quality
    Clubs
132 Brookline Ave.
Boston, MA 02115

A monthly magazine published exclusively for members of IRSA. Price included in membership.

Club Industry

Cardinal Business Media Inc.
1300 Virginia Drive, Suite 400
Fort Washington, PA 19044

A monthly business magazine for health and fitness facility management, providing an analysis of industry trends and happenings to more than 30,000 health and fitness professionals.

Council, The

Governor's Council on Physical
    Fitness and Sports
University of California,
    San Diego
9500 Gilman Drive
La Jolla, CA 92093

A quarterly, eight-page newsletter by the California Governor's Council on Physical Fitness &

Sports covering fitness, nutrition and sports news.

Exercise Standard, The

Super Slow Exercise Guild Inc.
P.O. Box 180154
Casselberry, FL 32718

A quarterly newsletter for fitness professionals. Topics include exercise physiology, programming, nutrition and general industry news. Price included in membership.

Exercise Standards and Malpractice Reporter, The

Professional Reports Corp.
4571 Stephens Circle N.W.
Canton, OH 44718

A bi-monthly newsletter on the legal aspects of exercise. $39.95/year.

ExerTrends

ExerTrends
800 Washington, Suite 309
Denver, CO 80203

Two monthly newsletters, one for clubs/facilities and the other for industry suppliers, providing current and unique research in psychological and physiological variables to understand existing and future market variables. Areas of study include equipment design and purchase, membership sales, advertising/marketing, developing new markets, membership retention and programming.

FDA Consumer

U.S. Superintendent of Documents
Washington, DC 20402-9371

The official magazine of the U.S. Food and Drug Administration, published 10 times a year, contains health articles and news related to food and drugs, such as investigations and court actions. $15/year.

Fitness Products Council Letter, The

Fitness Products Council
200 Castlewood Drive
North Palm Beach, FL 33408

A bi-monthly newsletter, published by the Fitness Products Council of the Sporting Goods Manufacturing Association, featuring fitness and nutrition information, research updates and trends. Free.

Harvard Business Review

Harvard University Graduate
School of Business Administration
P.O. Box 52623
Boulder, CO 80322

A bi-monthly educational journal for professional managers. $75/year.

ICHPER Journal

ICHPER
1900 Association Drive
Reston, VA 22091

The quarterly journal of the International Council for Health, Physical Education and Recreation, including sports students, health-related interviews, book reviews and more. Price included in membership.

IDEA Today

IDEA
The International Association
   for Fitness Professionals
6190 Cornerstone Court E.,
Suite 204
San Diego, CA 92121

Trade magazine published 10 times per year for exercise leaders. Price included in membership.

Issues in Food Safety

Issues in Food Safety
10866 Wilshire Blvd., Suite 550
Los Angeles, CA 90024

A quarterly, eight-page newsletter featuring food and safety news.

JAMA

American Medical Association
535 N. Dearborn St.
Chicago, IL 60610

The official weekly Journal of the American Medical Association. Price included in membership, $115/year nonmembers.

Journal Watch

Journal Watch
P.O. Box 9085
Waltham, MA 02254

A semi-monthly literature surveillance newsletter covering articles from major medical journals. $79/year.

Looking Fit

Virgo Publishing Inc.
4141 N. Scottsdale Road,
   Suite 316
Scottsdale, AZ 85251

The magazine for health-conscious tanning and toning centers. $54/year.

MACNews

Mid-Atlantic Club Management
   Association
12040 S. Lakes Drive
Reston, VA 22091

A quarterly newsletter covering association news. Price included in membership.

Medicine and Science in Sports and Exercise

MSSE, c/o Williams & Wilkins
P.O. Box 64380
Baltimore, MD 21264

The official journal of ACSM, featuring original investigations, clinical studies and comprehensive reviews on current topics in sports medicine. Published monthly. Free to members; $94/year nonmembers.

Muscle Media 2000

Muscle Media 2000
P.O. Box 277
Golden, CO 80402

A magazine covering bodybuilding issues. Published eight times per year. $36/year.

NSCA Bulletin

National Strength and
   Conditioning Association
P.O. Box 38909
Colorado Springs, CO 80937

A bi-monthly newsletter for NSCA members discussing association activities and developments. Price included in membership.

Network

Network Australia
P.O. Box 57
Neutral Bay, NSW 2089

A bi-monthly publication of Network For Fitness Professionals, covering programming, exercise physiology, product reviews, profiles and research updates. Price included in membership.

New England Journal of Medicine

Massachusetts Medical
   Society
10 Shattuck St.
Boston, MA 02115

A weekly journal of original research case studies and editorials in medicine and surgery. $99/year.

Olympian, The

U.S. Olympic Society
P.O. Box 1988
Boston, MA 02118

A magazine containing features, news and promotions by the U.S. Olympic Committee. Published 10 times per year. Price included in membership.

Peak Performance

United Research
1020 108th Ave. N.E., Suite 200
Bellevue, WA 98004

An eight-page, bi-weekly marketing research newsletter for health and athletic clubs. Included are two marketing reports, as well as a health and suppliers guide. $189/year.

Phil Kaplan's Health & Wealth Newsletter

Personal Development Services
1304 S.W. 160 Ave., Suite 337
Ft. Lauderdale, FL 33326

A monthly newsletter featuring marketing strategies for fitness products and services.

Physician & Sportsmedicine Journal, The

McGraw-Hill Healthcare Group
4530 W. 77th St.
Minneapolis, MN 5543

A monthly journal for physicians and sportmedicine specialists, including research, reviews, case reports and news. $46/year.

Pool & Spa News

Leisure Publications
3923 W. 6th St.
Los Angeles, CA 90020

Published 25 times per year with news, business and technical articles on the design, sales, building and maintenance of pools and spas. $17.97/year industry; $55/year nonindustry.

President's Council on Physical Fitness & Sports Newsletter

President's Council on Physical Fitness & Sports
450 5th St. N.W., Suite 7103
Washington, DC 20001

A bi-monthly newsletter covering youth fitness news. Free.

Priorities

American Council on Science and Health Inc.
1995 Broadway, 16th Floor
New York, NY 10023

A quarterly magazine by this non-profit consumer-education association, covering peer-reviewed reports on health and environmental issues, including scientifically balanced evaluations on nutrition, chemicals, lifestyle factors, the environment and human health. Price included in membership.

Running & Fitnews

American Running & Fitness Association
9310 Old Georgetown Road
Bethesda, MD 20814

An eight-page, monthly newsletter than covers health and fitness research. $25/year.

Self

Condé Nast Publications Inc.
350 Madison Ave.
New York, NY 10017.

A monthly magazine for women featuring the latest fitness, fashion, nutrition and health news. $15/year.

SGMA Today

SGMA
200 Castlewood Drive
North Palm Beach, FL 33408

A newsletter published 5 times per year for members of the Sporting Goods Manufacturers Association. Price included in membership.

Sports Medicine Bulletin

ACSM Public Information Department
P.O. Box 1440
Indianapolis, IN 46206

A quarterly newsmagazine for ACSM membership focusing on ACSM issues, activities, members, committees, regional chapter meetings, sports medicine conferences and meetings worldwide. Price included in membership.

Strength & Conditioning

National Strength and Conditioning Association
916 ROS St.
Lincoln, NE 68508

A bi-monthly journal featuring strength-conditioning methods and scientific and medical studies. Price included in membership.

University of California at Berkeley Wellness Letter

Health Letter Associates
P.O. Box 420176
Palm Coast, FL 32142

A monthly, eight-page consumer newsletter covering the latest findings and practice information on achieving a healthier wellness life. Includes topics such as nutrition, fitness and stress management. $24/year.

Vie

Vie Magazine
P.O. Box 6909
Marietta, GA 30065

A bi-monthly magazine distributed through clubs to its members featuring breakthroughs in exercise theory and application. $18/year.

Workplace Health

Workplace Health
8080 N. Central, LB78
Dallas, TX 75206

A monthly newsletter providing management, health and wellness ideas, and tips for employee managers, $120/year.

Books

America's Best Hoax: How doctors get fat on fitness

Book World
1933 Whitfield Loop
Sarasota, FL 34243

John LeMarr, 152pp, $12.95, 1994.

Balancing Act, The: Nutrition & weight guide

Balancing Act Nutrition
   Books
P.O. Box 671281
Dallas, TX 75367

Georgia G. Kostas, 320pp, $29.95, 1993.

Be Strong: Strength training for muscular fitness for men and women

Wm. C. Brown Publishers
2460 Kerper Blvd.
Dubuque, IA 52001

Wayne Westcott, 143pp, $15.22, 1993.

Body, Mind and Sport

Harmony Books
201 E. 50th St.
New York, NY 10022

John Douillard, 272pp, $22, 1994.

Business Planning Guide, The

Upstart Publishing Co.
12 Portland St.
Dover, NH 03820

David H. Bangs Jr., 184pp, $19.95, 1992.

Cross Training: Combining sports for exciting, balanced total-body workouts

Longmeadow Press
201 High Ridge Road
Stamford, CT 06904

R.G. "Nick" McNickle, 300pp, $12.95, 1994.

Design for Dignity

John Wiley & Sons Inc.
605 Third Ave.
New York, NY 10158

William L. Lebovich, 253pp, $4.95, 1993.

Don't Eat Your Heart Out Cookbook

Workman Publishing
708 Broadway
New York, NY 10003

Joseph C. Piscatella, 664pp, $17.95, 1994.

Essentials of Strength Training and Conditioning

Human Kinetics
P.O. Box 5076
Champaign, IL 61825

Thomas R. Baechle (ed.), 544pp, $45, 1994.

Exer-Deck: A guide to physical and recreation activity to enhance your health

Cardiovascular Health Program
Colorado Department of Public
   Health and Environment
4300 Cherry Creek Drive S.
Denver, CO 80222

Cardiovascular Disease Prevention Coalition, 82pp, $12, 1994 (4th ed.).

Exercise a la Carte: An activity menu to a healthier lifestyle

CVT Productions Inc.
440 Charnelton, Suite 220
Eugene, OR 97401

George L. Dixon Jr., 142pp, $12.95, 1994.

Exercise Empowerment Conditioning Cards: Abdominal exercises that work! Buns and leg exercises that work!

Debbie Reichenbach's Creative
   Concepts
2504 Caddy Lane
Joliet, IL 60435

Debbie Reichenbach's Creative Concepts, $7.95 each, 1994.

Exercise Handouts for Rehabilitation

Aspen Publishers
200 Orchard Ridge Drive,
   Suite 200
Gaithersburg, MD 20878

Carole B. Lewis & Therese McNerney, 515pp, $74, 1993.

Exercise in the Clinical Management of Diabetes

Human Kinetics
P.O. Box 5076
Champaign, IL 61825

Barbara N. Campaigne & Richard M. Lampman, 211pp, $32, 1994.

Fat Burning Diet, The: Accessing unlimited energy for a lifetime

Jay Robb Enterprises
Box 711533
Santee, CA 92072

Jay Robb, 138pp, $9.95, 1994.

Fit & Well: Core concepts and labs in physical fitness and wellness

Mayfield Publishing Co.
1280 Villa St.
Mountain View, CA 94041

Thomas D. Fahey, Paul M. Insel & Walton T. Roth, 280pp, $24.95, 1994.

Fitness Book, The: For people with disabilities

American Diabetes Association
1660 Duke St.
Alexandria, VA 22314

American Diabetes Association, 149pp, $14.95, 1994.

Fitness Cross-Training

Human Kinetics
P.O. Box 5076
Champaign, IL 61825

John Yacenda, 160pp, $14.95, 1994.

Fitness Instructor's Source Book, The

Debbie Reichenbach's Creative
    Concepts
2504 Caddy Lane
Joliet, IL 60435

Roy E. Vartabedian & Kathy Matthews, 120pp, $19.95, 1994 (2nd ed.).

Fitness Weight Training

Human Kinetics
P.O. Box 5076
Champaign, IL 61825

Thomas R. Baechle & Roger W. Earle, 160pp, $14.95, 1994.

Functional Rehabilitation in Orthopaedics

Aspen Publishers Inc.
200 Orchard Ridge Drive
Gaithersburg, MD 20878

Trudy Sandler Goldstein, 262pp, $58, 1995.

Health and Fitness Through Physical Education

Human Kinetics
P.O. Box 5076
Champaign, IL 61825

Russell R. Pate & Richard C. Hohn (eds.), 240pp, $38.95, 1994.

Health Promotion For All: Strategies for reaching diverse populations at the workplace

Wellness Councils of America
Community Health Plaza,
    Suite 311
7101 Newport Ave.
Omaha, NE 68152

Stephen Ramirez, 144pp, $25, 1994.

Health Robbers, The: A close look at quackery in America

Prometheus Books
59 John Glenn Drive
Amherst, NY 14228

Stephen Barrett & William T. Jarvis (eds.), 526pp, $35.95, 1993.

Hiring Right: A practical guide

Sage Publications
P.O. Box 5084
Thousand Oaks, CA 91359

Susan J. Herman, 177pp, $17.95, 1994.

How Consumers View Health and Sports Clubs

The University of Michigan
401 Washtenaw Ave.
Ann Arbor, MI 48109

Christine Brooks, 132pp, 1994.

How to Create Powerful Ads to Attract New Members: Modern day procedures for increasing the effectiveness of your promotions and advertising

Epoch Consultants Inc.
1220 Turner St., Suite F,
Clearwater, FL 34616

Klaus Hilgers & James Valko, 50pp, $145, 1992.

How to Prevent Falls

St. Martin's Press
175 Fifth Ave.
New York, NY 10010

Betty Perkins-Carpenter, 98pp, $8.95, 1993.

How to Start, Run and Stay in Business

John Wiley & Sons
605 Third Ave.
New York, NY 10158-0012

Gregory F. Kishel & Patricia Gunter Kishel, 222pp, $12.95, 1993.

HPER—Moving toward the 21st century

Human Kinetics
P.O. Box 5076
Champaign, IL 61825

Pat Duffy, Liam Dugdale (eds.), 352pp, $60, 1994.

Ideas for Action: Award winning approaches to physical activity

Sporting Goods Manufacturers
    Association
200 Castlewood Drive
North Palm Beach, FL 33408

SGMA, 200pp, $10, 1994.

Ins and Outs of Medical Insurance Billing, The

Medical Health and Fitness
P.O. Box 29
Santa Barbara, CA 93102

Eric P. Durak & Andrew A. Shapiro, 94pp, $39.95, 1994.

Introduction to Physical Education, Fitness and Sport

Mayfield Publishing Co.
1280 Villa St.
Mountain View, CA 94041

Daryl Siedentop, 385pp, $37.95, 1994 (2nd ed.).

Kinanthropometry in Aquatic Sports

Human Kinetics
P.O. Box 5076
Champaign, IL 61825

J.E. Lindsay Carter, Timothy R. Ackland (eds.), 174pp, $34.95, 1994.

Management Strategies in Athletic Training

Human Kinetics
P.O. Box 5076
Champaign, IL 61825

Richard Ray, 280pp, $42.95, 1994.

Managing Health Promotion Programs

Human Kinetics
P.O. Box 5076
Champaign, IL 61825

Bradley R.A. Wilson & Timothy E. Glaros, 264pp, $38, 1994.

Managing Stress: Principles and strategies for health and wellbeing

Jones & Bartlett Publishers
One Exeter Plaza
Boston, MA 02116

Brian Luke Seaward, 394pp, $32.50, 1994.

Max O₂

Health for Life
8033 Sunset Blvd., Suite 483
Los Angeles, CA 90046

Jerry Robinson & Frank Carrino, 210pp, $19.95, 1993.

Meltdown! Diet and Cookbook

Writers B-L-O-C-K
8216 Club Meadows Drive
Dallas, TX 75243

Beth Ellyn Rosenthal, 130pp, $15, 1994.

Natural Health Secrets From Around the World

Shot Tower Books
150 E. Palmetto Park Road, Suite 320
Boca Raton, FL 33432

Glenn W. Geelhoed, Robert D. Willix & Jean Barilla, 415pp, $24.95, 1994.

Necessary Toughness

American Diabetes Association
1660 Duke St.
Alexandria, VA 22314

Jonathan Hayes & Robert L. Briggs, 116pp, 1993.

Nutripoints: A new guide to simple, healthy eating

Designs for Wellness Press
P.O. Box 1450
Loma Linda, CA 92354

Roy E. Vartabedian & Kathy Matthews, 608pp, $9.95, 1994.

On the Guard II: The YMCA Lifeguard Manual

Human Kinetics
P.O. Box 5076
Champaign, IL 61825

YMCA, 232pp, $16, 1994 (2nd ed.).

PacifiCare's Health & Wellness Guide

PacifiCare
5701 Katella Ave.
Cypress, CA 90630

Karen S. Behnke & Robert Antonacci, 98pp, $10, 1994.

Personal Trainer Business Handbook, The

Willow Creek Publications
P.O. Box 86032
Gaithersburg, MD 20886

Ed Gaut, 136pp, $24.95, 1994.

Physical Activity, Fitness, and Health

Human Kinetics
P.O. Box 5076
Champaign, IL 61825

Claude Bouchard, Roy J. Shephard & Thomas Stephens, 1080pp, $128.50, 1994.

Physical Fitness: The hub of the wellness wheel

Kendall/Hunt Publishing Co.
4050 Westmark Drive
Dubuque, IA 52002

Bradley J. Cardinal, J.V. Krause, Mary E. Drabbs, 232pp, $19.16, 1992 (2nd ed.).

Physiology of Sport and Exercise

Human Kinetics
P.O. Box 5076
Champaign, IL 61825

Jack H. Wilmore & David L. Costill, 550pp, $49, 1994.

Polar Fat Free and Fit Forever Program, The

Fireside
1230 Avenue of the Americas
New York, NY 10020

James M. Rippe & Karla Dougherty, 160pp, $14.95, 1994.

Power Tennis Training

Human Kinetics
P.O. Box 5076
Champaign, IL 61825

Donald A. Chu, 160pp, $14.95, 1994.

Selecting Strength Exercises

National Youth Sports Foundation
10 Meredith Circle
Needham, MA 02192.

Wayne L. Westcott, 7pp, $5.25, 1993.

Selling Fitness: The complete guide to selling health club memberships

Communications Consultants
33 Knowles St.
Lincoln, RI 02865

Casey Conrad, 152pp, $29.95, 1994.

Senior Wellness Guide

Execu-Fit Health Programs
1 Lombard
San Francisco, CA 94111

Karen S. Behnke & Robert Antonacci, 102pp, $10, 1994.

Ski Energy: Alpine ski conditioning

Suzanne M. Nottingham Inc.
P.O. Box 710
Mammoth Lakes, CA 93546

Suzanne Nottingham, 50pp, $12, 1993.

Slim Forever

Sunshine Publications
P.O. Box 3669
Paramatta NSW 2124 Australia
Robert Harris, 310pp, $14.95, 1993.

Sports and Recreation for the Disabled

Cooper Publishing Group
701 Congressional Blvd.,
  Suite 340
Carmel, IN 46032
Michael J. Paciorek & Jeffery A. Jones, 424pp, $45, 1994 (2nd ed.).

Starting Your Own Business

McGraw Hill Inc.
1221 Avenue of the Americas
New York, NY 10020
Stephen C. Harper, 203pp, 1991.

Statistics in Kinesiology

Human Kinetics
P.O. Box 5076
Champaign, IL 61825
William J. Vincent, 280pp, $24, 1994.

Strength and Power in Sport

Human Kinetics
P.O. Box 5076
Champaign, IL 61825
P.V. Komi (ed.), 404pp, $39.95, 1992.

**Teaching Children Dance: Becoming a Master Teacher
Teaching Children Fitness: Becoming a Master Teacher
Teaching Children Games: Becoming a Master Teacher
Teaching Children Gymnastics: Becoming a Master Teacher
Teaching Children Movement Concepts and Skills: Becoming a Master Teacher**

Human Kinetics
P.O. Box 5076
Champaign, IL 61825
$14 each or $59 series, 1994.

The Comprehensive Guide to Work Injury Management

Aspen Publishers Inc.
200 Orchard Ridge Drive
Gaithersburg, MD 20878
Susan J. Isernhagen, 821pp, $75, 1995.

The Society of Prospective Medicine Handbook of Health Risk Appraisals

The Society of Prospective
  Medicine
4417 Anchor Mill Drive
Omaha, NE 68123
Kent W. Peterson & Sumner Brown Hiles (eds.), 265pp, $39.50, 1994.

Therapeutic Exercises Using the Swiss Ball

Executive Physical Therapy
P.O. Box 18864
Boulder, CO 80308
Caroline Corning Creager, 292pp, $39.95, 1994.

Toward Active Living

Human Kinetics
P.O. Box 5076
Champaign, IL 61825
H. Arthur Quinney, Lise Gauvin & A.E. Ted Wall (eds.), 312pp, $52.50, 1994.

Water Fitness During Your Pregnancy

Human Kinetics
P.O. Box 5076
Champaign, IL 61825
Jane Katz, 234pp, $17.95, 1994.

What's Cooking at the Cooper Clinic: Our best recipes for your best health

Jumbo Jack's Cookbooks
P.O. Box 247
Audubon, IA 50025
Cooper Clinic, 228pp, $14.95, 1992.

Women and Sport: Interdisciplinary perspectives

Human Kinetics
P.O. Box 5076
Champaign, IL 61825
D. Margaret Costa & Sharon R. Guthrie (eds.), 399pp, $60.50, 1994.

Worksite Health Promotion Economics: Consensus and analysis

Human Kinetics
P.O. Box 5076
Champaign, IL 61825
Robert L. Kaman (ed.), 256pp, $32, 1994.

YMCA Healthy Back Book

Human Kinetics
P.O. Box 5076
Champaign, IL 61825
Patricia Sammann, 110pp, $10.95, 1994.

Trade and Professional Associations

Aerobic Pipeline Int'l

3617 Drakeshire Dr.
Modesto, CA 95356
209 576-2611
Vicki Bretthauer, Exec. Dir.

International aerobic certification, personal training certification, choreography and floorwork workshops (ACE & AFAA credits) brought to clubs with groups of at least 15. Information packet and training site application available.

Aerobics & Fitness Association of America

15250 Ventura Blvd., Ste. 200
Sherman Oaks, CA 91403
800 445-5950 Fax 800 446-2322
Linda Pfeffer, R.N., Pres.

Multi-national organization for certification and education of aerobic exercise professionals and fitness leaders; also publishes American Fitness magazine, textbooks and study guidelines.

Amateur Athletic Union of the United States, Inc. (AAU)

AAU House
3400 W. 86th St.
P.O. Box 68207
Indianapolis, IN 46268
317 872-2900
Dr. Louis Marciani, Exec. Dir.

Amateur multi-sport organization.

American Academy of Pediatrics

141 N. West Point Blvd.
Box 927
Elk Grove Village, IL 60009-0927
708 228-5005
Crystal A. Milazzo, Project Mgr.

American Academy of Podiatric Sports Medicine (AAPSM)

1729 Glastonberry Rd.
Potomac, MD 20854
800 438-3355
Larry Shane, Exec. Dir.

AAPSM coordinates the various disciplines of podiatry, including podiatric medicine, biomechanics, surgery and physical therapy in the treatment of athletes. Membership requirements: a degree from an accredited college or university in podiatric medicine, physical education or biology.

American Association of Cardiovascular and Pulmonary Rehabilitation

7611 Elmwood Ave., Ste. #201
Middleton, WI 53562
608 831-6989
Alice Holbrow, Dir. Mktg.

American Athletic Trainers Association and Certification Board, Inc.

660 W. Duarte Rd.
Arcadia, CA 91007
818 445-1978
Joe S. Borland, R.P.T., C.S.M.T., Chm. Bd.

American College of Occupational & Environmental Medicine

55 W. Seegers Rd.
Arlington Hts., IL 60005
708 228-6850
D.I. Hoops, Ph.D.

An organization dedicated to promoting the health of workers through clinical practice, research and teaching.

American College of Sports Medicine (ACSM)

P.O. Box 1440
Indianapolis, IN 46206-1440
317 637-9200 Fax 317 634-7817
Susan L. Nelson, Dir. Public Information

The largest and oldest sports medicine and exercise science association in the world, with more than 14,000 members involved with medicine, science, education and allied health.

American Council On Exercise (ACE)

5820 Oberlin Dr.
San Diego, CA 92121-3787
619 535-8227
Sheryl Brown, Exec. Dir.

ACE is a not-for-profit, internationally recognized organization committed to enriching quality of life through safe and effective physical activity. ACE accomplishes its mission by setting certification standards for fitness instructors and, through public education and research.

American Diabetes Association

1660 Duke St.
Alexandria, VA 22314
703 549-1500
John H. Graham IV, C.E.O.

Organization supporting diabetes research and education. Founded in 1940 as a professional society, the ADA is an internationally recognized organization of affiliates and chapters in over 800 communities.

American Heart Association

7320 Greenville Ave.
Dallas, TX 75231
214 373-6300

American Medical Equestrian Assoc.

103 Surrey Rd.
Waynesville, NC 28786
704 456-3392
J.W. Thomas Byrd, M.D.

The primary mission of the AMEA is to emphasize safe participation for the rider/caregiver while maintaining a sense of tradition in the horse community.

American Medical Soccer Association

3508 Cheshire Dr.
Birmingham, AL 35242-3100
205 991-6054
Robert M. Cosby, M.D., Pres.

American Medical Society for Sports Medicine (AMSSM)

7611 Elmwood Ave., Ste. 202
Middleton, WI 53562
608 831-4484
Sheila Endicott, Exec. Dir.

A society of sports medicine physicians.

American Medical Tennis Assoc.

2301 Waleska Rd.
Canton, GA 30114
800 326-2682
Dr. Al Evans, Exec. Dir.

American Osteopathic Academy of Sports Medicine (AOASM)

7611 Elmwood Ave., Ste. 201
Middleton, WI 53562
608 831-4400
Robin Brown

American Paralysis Association (APA)

500 Morris Ave.
Springfield, NJ 07081
201 379-2690 Fax 800 225-0292
Mitchell R. Stoller, Pres./C.E.O.

APA supports and encourages research to find a cure for paralysis caused by spinal cord injury and other central nervous system disorders.

American Running & Fitness Association

4405 East-West Hwy., Ste. 405
Bethesda, MD 20814-1621
301 913-9517 Fax 800 776-2732
Susan Kalish, Exec. Dir.

A non-profit, educational association of athletes and sports-medicine professionals educating the public about the benefits of a regular aerobic exercise program and healthful diet. Members get free medical advice from volunteer sports-medicine professionals, a subscription to "Running & FitNews," and discounts on exercise gear, equipment and publications.

American Society of Biomechanics (ASB)

Orthopaedic Biomechanics Lab,
2432 5B
University of Iowa
Iowa City, IA 52242
319 335-7528
Thomas D. Brown, Pres.

ASB's purpose is to provide a forum for discussing techniques and applications of mechanics and mechanical analysis to research problems in biological science, medicine, sports science, or ergonomics. The society has about 700 members, and holds an annual scientific meeting.

American Sport Education Program (ASEP)

P.O. Box 5076
Champaign, IL 61825-5076
800 747-5698
Karen Partlow, Nat'l Dir.

ASEP (formerly the American Coaching Effectiveness Program) provides coaches, parents, and sport administrators with high-quality, research-based educational resources through three curriculums-SportCoach, SportParent, and SportDirector. ASEP is America's leading provider of sport education training and resources.

American Sports Education Institute/Boosters Club of America

200 Castlewood Dr.
North Palm Beach, FL 33408
407 842-3600
Michael May, Exec. Dir.

The national organization of fund-raising ideas for this country's high school booster clubs and youth sports programs.

American Youth Soccer Organization

5403 W. 138th St.
Hawthorne, CA 90250
310 643-6455
Dick Wilson, Nat'l Exec. Dir.

AYSO is a national non-profit organization dedicated to child development through youth soccer. Its "everyone plays...balanced teams...character counts" philosophies stress positive values, healthy exercise and education. AYSO has a nation-wide membership of 500,000 children and 250,000 volunteers.

Aquatic Exercise Association

P.O. Box 1609
Nokomis, FL 34274-1609
813 483-8600
Tracy Fryer

Networking and training organization for aquatic exercise professionals and aquatic therapists.

Association for the Advancement of Health Education

1900 Association Dr.
Reston, VA 22091
703 476-3437
Mary Hundley, Admin. Asst.

Association for Worksite Health Promotion

60 Revere Dr., Ste. 500
Northbrook, IL 60062
708 480-9574 Fax 708-480-9282
Valerie Powley, Membership
  Dir.

A membership society for work-site health professionals. Regional and local chapters offer networking opportunities. Student membership available.

Athletic Health Care System

Div. Sports Medicine
GB-15, University of Washington
Seattle, WA 98195
206 543-6734 Fax 206 543-6573
Stephen G. Rice, M.D.

Comprehensive system to prevent and manage athletic injuries.

Back to Work Rehabilitation Center

241 King St.
Northampton, MA 01060
413 586-2300
Nancy Caron

Boy Scouts of America

P.O. Box 152079
Irving, TX 75015-2079
214 580-2065
Richard Christian, Assoc. Dir.
   Employee Relations

In-house corporate fitness center and wellness program for employees only.

Canadian Academy of Sport Medicine

1600 James Naismith Dr.
Gloucester, ON
K1B 5N4
613 748-5851
Prog. Coord.

Canadian Association for Health, Physical Education, Recreation and Dance

1600 James Naismith Dr.,
Ste. 809
Gloucester, ON K1B 5N4
613 748-5622
Veronique Duvieusart, Dir.
Finance & Administration

Canadian Athletic Therapists Assoc. (CATA)

1600 James Naismith Dr.,
Ste. 507
Gloucester, ON K1B 5N4
613 748-5876
Mario Mercier, Pres.

Canadian Fitness & Lifestyle Research Institute

201-185 Somerset West
Ottawa, ON K2P 0J2
613 233-5528 Fax 613 233-5536
Angele Beaulieu, Commun.
   Officer

The Institute funds and initiates research on physically active lifestyles and communicates research knowledge to policymakers, professionals, and the general public.

Canadian Society for Exercise Physiology

1600 James Naismith Dr.,
Ste. 311
Gloucester, ON K1B 5N4
613 748-5768 Fax 613 748-5763
Bill Hearst, Exec. Dir.

Society for exercise physiology, health and fitness researchers.

Chicago School of Massage Therapy

2918 N. Lincoln Ave.
Chicago, IL 60657
312 477-9444
Robert King, Co-Dir.

Club Managers Association of America

1733 King St.
Alexandria, VA 22314
703 739-9500
Tamara J. Tyrrell

5,000-member professional association that represents managers of private golf, country, city, athletic, yacht, university and military clubs.

Cooper Institute for Aerobics Research

12330 Preston Rd.
Dallas, TX 75230
214 701-8001
Marilu Meredith

East Coast Alliance

64 Franklin Blvd.
Long Beach, NY 11561
516 432-6877 Fax 516 432-7044
Carol Lapidus-Scott

A non-profit organization for fitness professionals dedicated to providing quality education and networking opportunities, including newsletters, seminars, workshops and conventions.

Exercise & Sport Research Institute

Arizona State University
Tempe, AZ 85287
602 965-0040 Fax 602 965-7413
James S. Skinner, Ph.D., Dir.

An interdisciplinary institute for the study of human performance. Sections on biomechanics, exercise physiology and motor behavior/sport psychology.

Fitness Connection, The

11209 S. Grove St.
Huntley, IL 60142
708 669-0181
Pat Bieszki, Pres.

A nationwide training & educational service, providing quality certification and continuing education credit workshops from nationally recognized presenters and industry leaders to over 17,000 health clubs and fitness professionals across the U.S.

Hockey Development Centre for Ontario

Hockey Trainers' Certification
   Program
1185 Eglinton Ave. E., Ste. 301
Toronto, ON M3C 3C6
416 495-4060
John M. Panethere, Safety and
   Research Coordinator

IDEA, The Int'l Assoc. of Fitness Professionals

6190 Cornerstone Ct. E.,
Ste. 204
San Diego, CA 92121
619 535-8979
Communications Dept.

IDEA, the international association of fitness professionals, is the world's leading provider of continuing education and services for fitness professionals. Members include more than 23,000 fitness instructors, directors and personal trainers, as well as club and studio managers and owners in 72 countries around the world.

Industrial Athlete, The

116 Foxboro Dr.
Rochester Hills, MI 48309
313 375-2632
Dwight Gaal, C.E.O.

Management of on-site employee fitness, wellness and physical rehabilitation facilities. Will offer educaitonal programs for medical, physical rehabilitation and fitness professionals in 1995. Will also release a book in 1995 explaining the application of the "sports medicine model" of healthcare to the industrial setting.

International Council for Health, Physical Education, Recreation, Sport and Dance (ICHPER.SD)

1900 Association Dr.
Reston, VA 22091
703 476-3486
Dr. Dong Ja Yang

ICHPER.SD is dedicated to the scholarly pursuit and exchange of professional information among its members, all of whom are engaged in health, physical education, recreation, sport, dance or other related fields. ICHPER.SD has conducted biennial World Congresses since 1958.

International Council of Motorsport Sciences

8483 E. County Rd. 300 S
Plainfield, IN 46168
317 838-5888
Ms. Rusty Keifer, Exec. Secy.

International Health, Racquet and Sportsclub Assoc. (IHRSA)

263 Summer St.
Boston, MA 02210
800 228-4772 Fax 617 951-0055
John McCarthy, Exec. Dir.

A not-for-profit trade association for racquet, athletic and fitness clubs. Membership currently includes over 2400 clubs in 35 countries worldwide. Associate members—companies that sell products and services to the clubs—number 350. IHRSA also holds international conventions and trade shows twice a year.

International Institute for Sport & Human Performance

University of Oregon
1243 Bowerman Bldg.
Eugene, OR 97403
503 346-4114
Dr. Henriette Heiny, Dir.

Mission is to provide national and international markets with research results in the form of theses, dissertations and selected research publications (microfiche format) in the interrelated fields of exercise and sport sciences, physical education, health, fitness, leisure and dance.

International Kids' Fitness Association

12708 Catriona Ct.
Richmond, VA 23233
804 360-4285
Karen Armstrong, Dir.

An educational member-driven organization for fitness professionals who work with children. We provide the latest research and product information on this special population and provide a national certification program for fitness professionals who concentrate in the kids' fitness industry.

International Physical Fitness Association

415 W. Court St.
Flint, MI 48503
810 239-2166 Fax 810 239-9390
Jerry Kahn, Pres.

International School of Aerobic Training

6540 Lusk Blvd., Ste. C 214
San Diego, CA 92121
619 535-8283 Fax 619 535-9122
Ginger Banta, Director

For over 15 years ISAT has been bringing professional trainers to sites throughout the world. Courses are available in 7 languages, and their graduates are now top instructors in 27 countries. ISAT certification requires both written and performance examinations. Aerobic Instructor-60 hours. Personal Trainer-5 days. Step Instructor-4 days.

International Spa & Fitness Association

1300 "L" St. N.W., #1050
Washington, DC 20005
202 789-5920
Wayne J. Smith

The association serves as a clearinghouse of information on spa resorts, products and services. Members are provided training and marketing services, access to job opportunities and discounts on group purchasing of product and services.

International Sports Sciences Association

3920-B State St.
Santa Barbara, CA 93105
800 892-4772
Frank Miele

International Weightlifting Association (IWA)

P.O. Box 444
Hudson, OH 44236
216 655-9644 Fax 216 528-0488
John K. Norton

Joint Commission on Sports Medicine & Science

Oklahoma State University
Hospital & Clinic
1202 Farm Rd.
Stillwater, OK 74708
405 744-7031
Donald L. Cooper, M.D. & Co-Chm. or Doug Slifka, N.A.I.A.

Establishes guidelines and standards in the field of sports injury prevention and care, and provides recommendations for rules and procedures to be used in athletic programs.

Lake Placid Sports Medicine Society

Box 327
Lake Placid, NY 12946
518 523-1530
Bradford Stephens, M.D., V.P.

Mid-Atlantic Club Management Association (MACMA)

12040 S. Lakes Dr.
Reston, VA 22091
703 264-5049
W. Brent Arnold, Exec. Dir.

MACMA is a growing professional network of over 150 quality athletic, health, fitness, racquet and sports clubs in the Mid-Atlantic region. It is the largest region of clubs in the U.S. and represents over 200,000 club members. It is dedicated to expanding members' opportunities for communication, discussion, education and training.

National Academy of Sports Medicine (NASM)

2434 N. Greenview Ave.
Chicago, IL 60614
312 929-5101
Kim Bardley

Personal trainer workshop & certification.

National Association for Fitness Certification

P.O. Box 25997
Fresno, CA 73729
800 452-2548
Lynn Michaels, Exec. Dir.

Nationally recognized, the NAFC is dedicated to providing information and services to aspiring and established fitness professionals. Its emphasis is on

providing safe, effective and motivational training based on scientific principles. Certifications include fitness leader, aerobic instructor, step-right instructor and personal fitness trainer.

National Association for Girls & Women in Sport

1900 Association Dr.
Reston, VA 22091
703 476-3450
Mary Alice Hill

A non-profit, educational organization designed to serve the needs of administrators, teachers, coaches, leaders and participants of sport programs for girls and women. Focuses on advocacy, leadership and coaching. A member of the American Alliance for Health, Physical Education, Recreation and Dance.

National Association for Sport & Physical Education

1900 Association Dr.
Reston, VA 22091
703 476-3410
Judith Young, Ph.D., Exec. Dir.

National Association of Fitness Equip. Dealers & Service Technicians

967 Somerset St., Bldg. 116
Watchung, NJ 07060
908 604-0799
Phil Kaplan, Dir.

An association developed to set quality-of-service standards that health club operators can expect to receive from their associates and members. The membership includes qualified and ethical equipment dealers, service technicians, manufacturers representatives and reconditioning companies. The association acts as a consumers' advocate, industry watchdog and better business

bureau with the goal of customer satisfaction.

National Association of Governor's Councils on Physical Fitness & Sports

201 S. Capital Ave., Ste. 560
Indianapolis, IN 46225
317 237-5630
Cindy Porteous, Exec. Dir.

National Association of Orthopaedic Nurses

East Holly Ave.
Box 56
Pitman, NJ 08071-0056
609 256-2310
Pat Reichart, Exec. Secy. or
    Fran Reynolds, Membership
    Secy.

The National Association of Orthopaedic Nurses is a professional organization of nurses whose mission is to advance the delivery of orthopaedic patient care through specialty nursing education, standards, research, and the promotion of the interests and image of its members.

National Athletic Trainers Association (NATA)

2952 Stemmons Fwy.
Dallas, TX 75247
800 879-6282

NATA is a voluntary individual membership organization dedicated exclusively to promoting the interests of the athletic training profession, to providing a variety of useful services to athletic trainers, and to serving as a resource for information about the practice and profession of athletic training.

National Center for Health Education

72 Spring St., #208
New York, NY 10012-4019
212 334-9470 Fax 212 334-9845
David J. Andrews, Pres.

Since 1975, the NCHE has extended the power and reach of education for health. Operating through a cadre of volunteer facilitators, NCHE implements its comprehensive school health curriculum, "Growing Healthy," now taught in 41 states to more than one million students.

National Collegiate Athletic Assn. Injury Surveillance System (ISS)

6201 College Blvd.
Overland Park, KS 66211
913 339-1906
Randall W. Dick, Asst. Dir.
   Sports Sciences

The ISS currently monitors injuries in 16 collegiate sports. Approximately 15% of schools sponsoring a particular sport participate annually, with the sampling accounting for regional and divisional distribution.

National Congress of PTA

330 N. Wabash Ave., Ste. 2100
Chicago, IL 60611-3690
312 670-6782
Kathyrn Whitfill, Pres.

National Council Against Health Fraud, Inc.

P.O. Box 1276
Loma Linda, CA 92354
909 824-4690 Fax 909 824-4838
Dr. William Jarvis

A non-profit organization comprised of health professionals, educators, researchers, attorneys and concerned citizens who actively oppose misinformation, fraud and quackery in the health marketplace. 1. Bimonthly newsletter available to members or subscribers. 2. Bimonthly Bulletin Board also mailed to members. 3. Position papers available. See "Available Resource Materials"-free upon

request. 4. "Recommended Anti-quackery Publications"-free upon request.

National Dance Association

1900 Association Dr.
Reston, VA 22091
703 476-3436 Fax 703 476-9527
Rebecca Hutton, Exec. Dir.

A service organization working with a national and international network of artists and arts educators to assess and enhance the quantity and quality of dance in schools, colleges, studios and other settings. Provides leadership in resource identification, publications, curriculum design, certification, advocacy and professional development.

National Dance-Exercise Instructor's Training Association

1503 Washington Ave. S.,
Ste. 208
Minneapolis, MN 55454
800 237-6242
Linda Benzinger

National aerobics training and certification organization. Conducts one-day certification and training workshops for aerobics and fitness instructors nationwide. Also has teacher training video programs for low-impact aerobics and new aerobic workouts. Now offering step certification also.

National Employee Services & Recreation Association

2211 York Rd., Ste. 207
Oakbrook, IL 60521-2371
708 368-1280
Patrick B. Stinson, Exec. Dir.

Serves organizations and individuals responsible for providing employee services, recreation and fitness/health programs through education,

information and professional development.

National Exercise for Life Institute (NEFLI)

P.O. Box 2000
Excelsior, MN 55331-9967
800 358-3636 Fax 612 368-2794
Kelly Stave

NEFLI encourages people to begin and maintain a personal exercise program by providing free educational materials, a toll-free fitness hotline, and a health professionals information & referral network, and by coordinating ongoing fitness research.

National Federation of Interscholastic Coaches Association

11724 Plaza Cir.
P.O. Box 20626
Kansas City, MO 64195
816 464-5400
Don Sparks, Dir.

Provides $1,000,000 liability insurance protection for coaches for a yearly fee. Membership also includes issues of the National Federation NEWS magazine and various hotel and car rental discounts.

National Football Head & Neck Injury Registry

Univ. of Pennsylvania, Sports
   Medicine Ctr.
Weightman Hall E-7, 235 S.
   33rd St.
Philadelphia, PA 19104
215 662-6943
Joseph S. Torg, M.D.

National Head Injury Foundation

1776 Massachusetts Ave. N.W.,
   Ste. 100
Washington, DC 20036
202 296-6443
Mary Reitter, Prog. Dir.

A national membership organization dedicated to improving the quality of life for persons with traumatic brain injury. For that cause, the Foundation conducts political advocacy, public and professional education and a variety of direct support programs. Included in its ranks are 44 state associations and hundreds of local support groups.

National Health Club Association

12596 W. Bayaud Ave., 1st Fl.
Denver, CO 80228
800 765-6422
Sean Kirby

The NHCA provides programs and services to help increase the value in your club's membership, lower operating costs and increase profitability. Programs and services include: business tracking & evaluation, a workout progress system, sales & management training, a weight management program, group medical & liability insurance, instructor certification and instructor liability insurance.

National Institute on Aging

Bldg. 31, Rm. 5C27
Bethesda, MD 20892
301 496-1752
Jane E. Shure, Info. Officer

NIA provides public and professional health information materials on frailty, exercise & aging and other biomedical, social and behavioral research on aging and the special needs of older people. For publications call 1-800-222-2225.

National Institutes of Health, Recreation & Welfare Assn.

9000 Wisconsin Ave.
Bldg. 31, B1W30
Bethesda, MD 20892
301 496-6061
Randy Schools, CAE

Fitness, recreation and employee services.

National Intramural-Recreational Sports Association (NIRSA)

850 S.W. 15th St.
Corvallis, OR 97333-4145
503 737-2088
Will M. Holsberry

Premier association for recreational sports professionals and their institutions. Publishes NIRSA Journal (three times annually), NIRSA Newsletter (quarterly), Recreational Sports Directory (annually), Outstanding Sports Facilities Directory, and program guides. Sponsors state and regional workshops, plus annual national conference and exhibit show.

National Recreation & Park Association

2775 South Quincy St., Ste. 300
Arlington, VA 22206
703 820-4940
R. Dean Tice, Exec. Dir.

NRPA is a not-for-profit, service, research and education organization, serving as the united voice of the park and recreation movement. NRPA is dedicated to the wise use of leisure time, conservation of our natural and human resources and beautification of the American environment. The association serves federal, state and local governments as well as private organizations and citizen efforts.

National Sporting Goods Association

1699 Wall St.
Mt. Prospect, IL 60056
312 439-4000
Daniel S. Kasen, Information Specialist

National Strength and Conditioning Association

P.O. Box 38909
Colorado Springs, CO 80937
719 632-6722
Membership Dept.

A non-profit, educational association promoting applied sport science research and its practical applications for the development of physical performance with reduced injury.

National Wellness Association

1045 Clark St., Ste. 210
P.O. Box 827
Stevens Pt., WI 54481-0827
715 342-3969
Anne Helmke, Dir. Memberships Svcs. & Health Prom.

A national resource center for wellness professionals. Mission is to collect and disseminate wellness information, to provide networking opportunities and to provide health promotion & wellness resources for members. Individual and organizational memberships. Benefits include: National Wellness Resource Directory; Wellness Management, a quarterly newsletter; Member Directory; Job Bulletin; conference and product discounts; Health Issues Update, quarterly newsletters.

National Youth Sports Foundation for the Prevention of Athletic Injuries

10 Meredith Cir.
Needham, MA 02192
617 449-2499
Rita Glassman, Assoc. Exec. Dir.

A non-profit (501 C3) educational research foundation that works to promote the safety and well-being of children and adolescents participating in sports. The foundation acts as an educational resource for

*program administrators,
coaches, parents, health professionals and athletes.*

NERSA, The New England Association of Quality Clubs

263 Summer St.
Boston, MA 02210
617 951-0055
Jan Woodman, Exec. Dir.

Office of Disease Prevention & Health Promotion

330 "C" St. S.W., Rm. 2132
Suitzer Bldg.
Washington, DC 20201
202 205-8611
Dr. J. Michael McGinnis, Dir.

*ODPHP coordinates policy and
program development in prevention for the Department of
Health & Human Services. Also
serves as the coordinating office for Healthy People 2000:
National Health Promotion
and Disease Prevention Objectives. Also answers inquiries
from the public & professionals,
and distributes material on
health information resources
through the ODPHP National
Health Information Center
(NHIC).*

Overeaters Anonymous, Inc.

6075 Zenith Ct., NE
Rio Rancho, NM 87124
505 891-2664
Jorge N. Sever, Exec. Dir.

Physical Medicine Research Foundation

207 W. Hastings St., Ste. 510
Vancouver, BC V6B 1H7
604 684-4148
Marc White, Exec. Dir.

*The foundation is committed to
improving the quality of life for
people suffering pain from physical injuries and dysfunction
through research, education,
and cooperation among all
health care practitioners.*

Physical Therapy Specialties

5990 Stoneridge Dr., Ste. 122B
Pleasanton, CA 94588
510 734-8005
Ida Hirst, R.P.T.

*Physical Therapy Specialities is
an outpatient physical therapy
center which offers treatment
for orthopaedic injuries resulting from work, athletic, au-
tomobile, or other accidents.
Programs emphasize therapeutic exercise to help regain mobil-
ity and strength.*

Physicians Information & Referral Network (PIRN)

P.O. Box 2000
Excelsior, MN 55331-9967
800 358-3636 Fax 612 368-2794
Kelly Stave

*PIRN connects health profession-
als to exchange information
and ideas about exercise/reha-
bilitation options. It also provides free educational
materials and current research
findings for counseling
patients/clients on exercise and
positively influencing lifestyle
habits.*

President's Council on Physical Fitness & Sports

701 Pennsylvania Ave. N.W.,
    Ste. 250
Washington, DC 20004-2608
202 272-3421
Sandra Perimatter, Exec. Dir.

Prevent Blindness America

500 E. Remington Rd.
Schaumburg, IL 60173-4556
800 331-2020
Tod W. Turiff, Dir. Programs

*Collects, analyzes and dissemi-
nates information and materials that can be used to prevent
or reduce morbidity from eye
trauma and to promote eye injury prevent strategies. Single
copies of materials provided
free of charge.*

Professional Fitness Instructor Training (PRO-FIT)

12012 156th Ave., S.E.
Renton, WA 98059-6317
206 255-3817
Alice Lockridge, M.S. Phys. Ed.

*PRO-FIT conducts fitness in-
structor training courses
throughout the year in the Seattle area. Products developed for
professional instructors are:
heart rate charts, personal
trainer contracts, nutritional
educational posters, anatomy t-
shirts and PRO-FACTS: Certification Study Cards, Flask Anatomy Muscle Study Cards &
Anatomy Academy Pronuncia-
tion Audio Tapes.*

Recreation Safety Institute

Box 392
Ronkonkoma, NY 11779
516 563-4806
Dr. Arthur Mittlestaedt, Jr.,
Ed.D, Exec. Dir.

*The non-profit membership
assoc. provides safety inspections, audits, certification of
products and other advocacy
projects.*

Resort & Commercial Recreation Association

P.O. Box 1208
New Port Richey, FL 34656
813 845-7373
Frank Oliveto, Exec. Dir.

Safety Resource Centre

Ontario Sports and Recreation
    Centre
1185 Eglinton Ave. E.
New York, Ontario, Canada
M3C 3C6
Nancy Singer

*Provides safety-related informa-
tion in the areas of sport, fitness and recreation.*

Society of Prospective Medicine

4417 Anchor Mill Dr.
Omaha, NE 68123
402 291-3297 Fax 402 293-1607
Janet Foerster, M.Ed.

An interdisciplinary society for the advancement of health promotion through health-risk assessment.

Special Olympics International

1325 "G" St. N.W., Ste. 500
Washington, DC 20005
202 628-3630
Edgar May, C.O.O.

Sporting Goods Agents Association

P.O. Box 998
Morton Grove, IL 60053
312 296-3670 Fax 708 827-0196
Lois Halinton, Exec. Dir.

International trade association of independent sporting goods agents.

Sports & Scan Cardiovascular Nutritionists (SCAN)

7730 E. Belleview Ave., G-6
Englewood, CO 80111
303 779-1950
Linda Newcomb or Nicki
    Zeidner, Chair

A dietetic practice group of the American Dietetic Association.

Sports Safety Board of Quebec

100 Laviolette Ave.
Bureau 114
Trois-Rivieres, Quebec, Canada
G9A 5S9
819 371-6033
Claude Goulet, Research
    Officer

Surfer's Medical Association

P.O. Box 1287
Aptus, CA 95001-1287
408 684-0916
Paula Smith

United States Association of Blind Athletes

33 N. Institute St.
Colorado Springs, CO 80903
719 630-0422 Fax 719 630-0616
Charlie Huebner, Exec. Dir. or
    Mark Lucas, Asst. Exec. Dir.

USABA is a non-profit organization dedicated to the development of individual independence through athletic competition for the blind/visually impaired. USABA is the official U.S. organization to train, coach, and prepare blind athletes for national competition in both winter and summer sports.

United States Racquet Stringers Association

P.O. Box 40
Del Mar, CA 92014
619 481-3545
Jill Workman, Exec. Dir.

USRSA was founded in 1975 to provide resource information for professional racquet stringers. Today, more than 6,000 of its members rely on the organization's technical expertise, product updates and equipment reviews on racquet strings, frames and stringing machines. The USRSA also offers members marketing assistance and a nationwide Stringer Certification Program.

United States Squash Racquets Association

P.O. Box 1216
Bala-Cynwyd, PA 19004
610 667-4006 Fax 610 667-6539
Craig W. Brand, Exec. Dir.

The governing body for squash in the U.S. Sets the game rules and equipment specifications, sanctions tournaments, ranks players and holds 83 national championships annually.

United States Water Fitness Association, Inc.

P.O. Box 3279
Boynton Beach, FL 33424-3279
407 732-9908
John R. Spannuth, Pres./C.E.O.

A national non-profit organization designed to promote water fitness, unite people and organizations to work together, certify instructors (basic & advanced), improve communications, design programs to increase participation and revenue, develop leadership, name the top water fitness facilities to improve their programs.

United States Weightlifting Federation

One Olympic Plaza
Colorado Springs, CO 80909-
    5764
719 578-4508
George Greenway, Exec. Dir.

National governing body for U.S. Olympic weightlifting. Selects international teams for events such as the World Championships, Pan Am and Olympic Games. Also promotes amateur weightlifting.

Washington Business Group on Health

777 N. Capitol St. N.E., Ste. 800
Washington, DC 20002
202 408-9320
Mary Hebert

Wellness Councils of America

Community Health Plaza
7101 Newport Ave., Ste. 311
Omaha, NE 68152-2175
402 572-3590 Fax 402 572-3594
Harold S. Kahler Jr., Ph.D.,
    Pres.

A national non-profit organization dedicated to promoting healthier lifestyles for all Americans, especially through health promotion activities at the worksite.

Wilderness Medical Society

P.O. Box 2463
Indianapolis, IN 46206-2463
317 631-1745
Warren Bowman, M.D., Pres.

The Wilderness Medical Society was established to provide a central organization to promote research and educational activities that increase medical knowledge about human activities in wilderness environments.

Women's Sports Foundation

Eisenhower Park
East Meadow, NY 11554
800 227-3988
Donna Lopiano, Ph.D., Exec. Dir.

A non-profit educational organization dedicated to enhancing and expanding fitness and sports experiences for all girls and women.

Young American Bowling Alliance

5301 S. 76th St.
Greendale, WI 53129-1192
414 421-4700 Fax 414 421-1301
Renee Schlitz, Commun. Mgr.

Personal Training Certifications

Aerobics and Fitness Association of America
15250 Ventura Blvd., Suite 200
Sherman Oaks, CA 91403-3297

Type: Personal Trainer/Fitness Counselor

Purpose: For the fitness professionals who work with clients on a one-on-one basis

Prerequisites: AFAA primary certification (for aerobics instructors) or successful completion of introduction course

Certification: Written and practical examinations; workshop is 3 days

American College of Sports Medicine
P.O. Box 1440
Indianapolis, IN 46206-1440

Type: Health Fitness Instructor

Purpose: Candidates must demonstrate competency in exercise fitness testing, designing and executing an exercise program, leading exercise, and operating a fitness facility

Prerequisites: Bachelor's degree in exercise science, physical education, or allied health

Certification: Written and practical examinations

American Council on Exercise
5820 Oberlin Drive, Suite 102
San Diego, CA 92121

Type: Personal Trainer

Purpose: For individuals working with clients on a one-on-one basis

Prerequisites: No advanced education is required, candidates must be 18 years of age and CPR certified

Certification: Written test only

Cooper Institute for Aerobics Research
12330 Preston Rd.
Dallas, TX 75230

Type: Physical Fitness Specialist

Purpose: To provide training of fitness leadership and technical skills necessary for the implementation of an individualized physical fitness program

Prerequisites: Must attend a 40-hour workshop

Certification: Written and practical examinations

National Strength
and Conditioning Association
CSCS Agency
P.O. Box 83469
Lincoln, NE 68501

Type: Personal Trainer Certification

Purpose: For professionals who train clients in a one-on-one situation in clients' homes, health/fitness clubs, and YMCAs.

Prerequisites: No postsecondary coursework or degree is required, but candidates must have a good working knowledge of biomechanical concepts, training adaptations, anatomy, exercise physiology, and program design guidelines

Certification: 120 multiple-choice questions, 30 of which correspond with 30 videotape segments; the videotape segments assess knowledge primarily in the exercise technique area

Canadian Society for Exercise Physiology
1600 James Naismith Dr., Ste. 311
Gloucester, ON K1B 5N4

Type: Certified Fitness Appraiser

Purpose: To recognize advanced preparation of fitness appraisers with formal training in exercise science and lifestyle counseling.

Prerequisites: CPR certification; undergraduate degree in exercise science or the equivalent; current STFA registration; completion of a FACA-sanctioned apprenticeship or workshop (contact the Canadian Society for Exercise Physiology for more information on STFA and FACA)

Certification: Written and practical examinations; annual recertification required

Index

P

About the Authors

Scott O. Roberts, MS, CSCS, received his BA in physical education from California State University, Chico; his MS in exercise physiology from California State University, Sacramento; and will soon receive his PhD from the University of New Mexico. He is a Certified Strength and Conditioning Specialist through the National Strength and Conditioning Association, and a Certified Exercise Program Director through the American College of Sports Medicine.

Scott is assistant professor of exercise and sport science at Texas Tech University. He also is president of Scott Roberts Enterprises, Ltd., a fitness education consulting company. He has received many recognitions, most recently being listed in the 1994-1995 edition of *Who's Who in American Education*. He is a frequent presenter at national sports medicine and fitness conferences. He has authored many research papers, articles, and books, including *Strength and Weight Training for Young Athletes*. Scott is married and has three children. In his spare time, he enjoys walking, mountain biking, and playing music.

Dr. **Kathy Alexander**, exercise physiologist and health promotion specialist, is the cofounder and CEO of S.T.E.P.S., Inc. (Scientific Training and Exercise Prescription Specialists), a personal training facility and consulting firm located in Nashville, TN. Dr. Alexander's clients have included Nissan Motor Manufacturing Co. and the Internal Revenue Service, and she has contributed to such publications as *Cooking Light Magazine*, *Mademoiselle*, and the *Washington Post*. She received both her bachelor's and master's degrees from the University of Tennessee-Knoxville, and her doctorate from Vanderbilt University. Dr. Alexander has taught exercise physiology and wellness-related courses at the university level.

Douglas Brooks, MS, exercise physiologist, received his master's degree in exercise physiology from Central Michigan University. He has been recognized by many publications as one of the country's premier personal trainers. Douglas frequently conducts lectures and workshops on exercise physiology, kinesiology, strength training, and personal training. He is the author of *Going Solo—The Art of Personal Training*, *Program Design for Personal Trainers*, and *Practical Fitness Testing and Assessment for Personal Trainers*. Douglas is a member of the advisory board for IDEA and works on the development team for Step Reebok programs. He has directed a 5,000-member health facility, actively participated in and coached college-level gymnastics, was an assistant professor in the health science department at the University of Michigan, and most recently owned and operated a personal training facility for 9 years. He is a competitive marathon runner and triathlete and an avid rock climber and mountaineer. Douglas lives in Mammoth Lakes, CA, with his wife Candice and their two sons.

Gregory J. Florez is president of First Fitness, Inc., a Chicago-based health and fitness company with operations in Illinois, Indianapolis, and Washington, D.C. First Fitness designs and equips commercial and residential fitness facilities and provides consulting and program design services, personal training, and many other wellness-related services. Gregory writes and lectures frequently for organizations such as the American College of Sports Medicine, IDEA, and several national consumer magazines. He is also on the staff of Personal Trainer Resources, an organization that provides educational materials and tools to personal trainers.

James Gavin has been a university professor and practicing psychologist since 1968, specializing in health promotion and counseling psychology. He earned his doctorate in psychology from New York University in 1969 and was awarded the Diplomate in Counseling Psychology by the American Board of Professional Psychology in 1984. Since 1980, Jim has been a professor of applied social science at Concordia University in Montreal. In keeping with his beliefs about health and fitness, Jim has been a competitive swimmer, triathlete, modern dancer, aerobics instructor, and yoga teacher.

Nettie Gavin has a private practice in body-mind integration therapy, specializing in holistic transformations. She earned her master's degree in public administration from the University of Pittsburgh in 1975 with a concentration in group dynamics. A student of healing arts since 1974, Nettie has studied transpersonal psychology, yoga, t'ai chi, aikido, meditation, polarity therapy, and Kripalu bodywork.

David L. Herbert received his BBA from Kent State University in 1971 and his JD from the University of Akron College of Law in 1974. He is a senior partner in the law firm of Herbert, Benson & Scott. Mr. Herbert has lectured at several universities and served as associate professor at Kent State University. He has made many presentations and keynote addresses to such groups as the American College of Sports Medicine and the National Strength and Conditioning Association. He is also president of PRC Publishing, Inc., publishers of periodicals dealing with malpractice, sports medicine, health care law, and many other topics. He is a member of the editorial review board for the journal *The Physician and Sportsmedicine*, among other journals, and writes regular columns for many others. He has been a consultant for several organizations such as the American College of Sports Medicine and the American Association for Cardiovascular and Pulmonary Rehabilitation. Mr. Herbert is also vice president of Medical Risk Management Services, Inc., an Ohio health care provider risk management company. He has authored many books and articles.

Amy T. Huggins is past owner and president of Well Beings, Inc., a business that provides training within corporations and professional organizations to promote fitness, stress management, and communications. Amy speaks regularly at fitness industry conventions, and has been a contributing author to several newsletters and books. She is gold-certified by the American Council on Exercise, and is certified in CPR by the Red Cross. Amy served as a lifestyle ambassador for the Rockport Company in 1990. In 1983, she received her master's degree in marketing from the J.L. Kellogg Graduate School of Management at Northwestern University.

Mark A. Reiff, MS, CSCS, received his bachelor's degree in mathematics and history from the University of Indianapolis in 1978, and his master's degree in exercise physiology from Indiana University in 1988. He is certified as a Level 1 Coach by the United States Weightlifting Association and as a Certified Strength and Conditioning Specialist by the National Strength and Conditioning Association (NSCA). He has held several offices in NSCA, including vice president and secretary-treasurer. Mark has had coaching positions at Yale University, California State University (Long Beach), and Stanford University.

Irv Rubenstein received his PhD in exercise sciences from Peabody College-Vanderbilt University. He is cofounder and president of S.T.E.P.S., Inc. He has a personal fitness trainer certification from the American Council on Exercise, is certified by the National Strength and Conditioning Association as a Certified Strength and Conditioning Specialist, and is certified by the American College of Sports Medicine as a Health and Fitness Instructor. Dr. Rubenstein is a personal trainer, and through S.T.E.P.S., Inc., provides seminars and consultations in exercise and wellness. He has also consulted with exercise equipment manufacturers on the design and implementation of their products.

David B. Rusk has been a personal trainer since 1986. He is certified through the National Strength and Conditioning Association and the American College of Sports Medicine. David's degree is from the College of Business Administration at the University of Cincinnati. His educational background, as well as 12 years of public and private accounting, were instrumental in equipping him to run his personal training business. He has spoken at the 1993 and 1994 National Strength and Conditioning Association national conferences and has written several articles for fitness magazines. David lives in Long Beach, CA.